ALL ABOUT EVE
Your Women's Health
Questions Answered

ALL ABOUT EVE
Your Women's Health
Questions Answered

Editors

Annabel Chew

Ho Ching Lin

Jade Kua

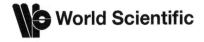

Association of Women
Doctors (Singapore)

World Scientific

Published by

World Scientific Publishing Co. Pte. Ltd.

5 Toh Tuck Link, Singapore 596224

USA office: 27 Warren Street, Suite 401-402, Hackensack, NJ 07601

UK office: 57 Shelton Street, Covent Garden, London WC2H 9HE

Library of Congress Cataloging-in-Publication Data
Names: Chew, Annabel, editor. | Ho, Ching Lin, editor. | Kua, Jade, editor.
Title: All about Eve : your women's health questions answered / editors,
    Annabel Chew, Ho Ching Lin, Jade Kua.
Description: New Jersey : World Scientific, [2022] | Includes bibliographical references and index.
Identifiers: LCCN 2021050511 | ISBN 9789811237799 (hardcover) |
    ISBN 9789811238536 (paperback) | ISBN 9789811237805 (ebook) |
    ISBN 9789811237812 (ebook other)
Subjects: LCSH: Women--Health and hygiene. | Women--Health and hygiene--Miscellanea. |
    Humanistic psychology.
Classification: LCC RA778 .A4385 2022 | DDC 613/.04244--dc23/eng/20211128
LC record available at https://lccn.loc.gov/2021050511

British Library Cataloguing-in-Publication Data
A catalogue record for this book is available from the British Library.

For any available supplementary material, please visit
https://www.worldscientific.com/worldscibooks/10.1142/12302#t=suppl

EDITORS' BIOGRAPHIES

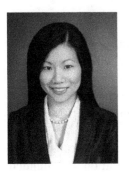 Dr Annabel Chew is a Senior Consultant of the Glaucoma department in the Singapore National Eye Centre. She holds various academic appointments; she is a Clinical Assistant Professor of Duke-NUS Graduate Medical School, and an Adjunct Clinician Investigator at the Singapore Eye Research Institute. Dr Chew is actively involved in postgraduate and undergraduate education of ophthalmology trainees and medical students, as well as paramedical staff, including optometrists and nurses. Dr Chew's current research interest is in glaucoma, and she has published scientific papers in respected peer-reviewed medical journals.

She is the Treasurer and immediate past Vice President of the Association of Women Doctors Singapore.

Association of Women
Doctors (Singapore)

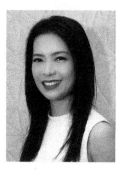

Clinical Associate Professor Ho Ching Lin is a Senior Consultant and immediate past Head of Glaucoma Service at the Singapore National Eye Centre. She is also the Director of Philanthropy and Development for the Eye academic clinical program of the Duke-NUS Graduate Medical School. She holds both a Paediatrics as well as Ophthalmology specialist degrees, is a Glaucoma and Paediatric Glaucoma specialist, and is visiting Senior Consultant at National University Hospital and KK Women's and Children's Hospital. She is the Director of the charity VisionSave, Chairman of the Eye Ball as well as the Eye Run and Cycle. She has been conferred several awards for her activities in charities, blindness prevention work and community service.

She is the immediate past President of the AWDS and this book was one of the projects she initiated during her term.

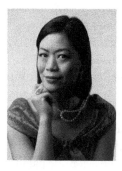

Dr Jade Kua is a senior consultant in general and pediatric emergency medicine, with a masters in trauma. She is a Past President of the Association of Women Doctors, Singapore and the immediate Past President of the Singapore Anti-Narcotics Association.

She is also a professional life coach accredited by the International Coaching Federation and founded Jade Life And Wellness. Her children's bedtime book on mindfulness, Good Night Marion, was published by Write Editions and used by therapists, psychologists and parenting experts.

Dr Seow Yian San, current President of the Association of Women Doctors Singapore, and Dr Gayathri Nadarajan, past Secretary of the Association of Women Doctors Singapore, are associate editors of the book.

FOREWORD

by the President of the Republic of Singapore

A book by female doctors addressing common female health problems is not only timely and relevant, but also extremely empowering. When women receive information about their health issues from female physicians with an intimate understanding of what they are going through, it allows them to make informed decisions which can positively impact other areas of their lives.

This book provides concise information on a whole range of topics on women's health and covers key issues across different stages of their lives such as adolescent health, family planning, pregnancy, breastfeeding, common gynaecological conditions, menopause, the psychological impact of ageing, end-of-life planning, and many more.

Since its registration in 1998, the Association of Women Doctors Singapore (AWDS) has successfully launched many barrier-breaking initiatives in promoting women's rights in relation to health and career advancement in medical practice. This book is yet another illustration of the extensive contributions of women in the medical field in Singapore, many of whom have also worked tirelessly in the fight against COVID-19.

I strongly believe in empowering women to make informed decisions about their health. I commend AWDS for producing this book to improve health literacy among women. This effort demonstrates the importance of a whole-of-society effort and community partnerships to empower, support and uplift our Singapore women. I hope you will use the knowledge gained from this book to invest in your well-being, and the well-being of the women around you.

Halimah Yacob
President of the Republic of Singapore

FOREWORD

by the Permanent Secretary (Communications &
Information), Singapore Civil Service

I greatly enjoyed reading this book *All about Eve: Your Women's Health Questions Answered*, produced by the Association of Women Doctors Singapore. It is a book written by our doctors in Singapore to address the common questions women have about our health conditions and our bodies, at different stages of our lives. It is written in language for the layman so that it can be easily understood, and it focuses on issues and questions we have.

All of us have questions about health conditions, whether our own or that of our loved ones or friends. The answers are usually found in multiple places and we may not always be sure about the credibility of the information in articles we might find, such as on the internet. Explanations may also be highly technical and not easy to understand. What's more, we often don't know what to ask, not to mention, whom to ask.

This is thus a valuable book because it brings together easy-to-understand answers for issues we have. I found the book very informative. Many people are fearful of what they don't understand. For me, the simply presented and clear explanations helped calm my fears and uncertainty. The well-written essays give clear medical explanations, written in ways to help the public understand the various conditions that women face and what we need to do. The organization of the 25 essays by stages of life is helpful to navigate the complex subject of healthcare. I also appreciated the thoughtful inclusion of some common, but difficult to raise, issues.

I commend the Association of Women Doctors Singapore and its many dedicated members for producing this book. Their combined efforts to write and edit essays to serve their audience reflect their commitment to their profession and care for their patients. Let me also thank the Singapore Council of Women's Organisations for their grant funding of this worthy project. I hope women of all ages will find reading the book as enjoyable and useful as I have.

Yong Ying-I
Permanent Secretary (Communications & Information)
and former Permanent Secretary (Health)
Singapore Civil Service

FOREWORD

It is health that is real wealth and not the pieces of gold and silver...

— Mahatma Gandhi

I've stared death in the face. But, death blinked first. It hasn't made me brave nor invincible. It has however made me realise even more that life is fleeting. My family claims we've won the biggest lottery because health is no different from money. Until we face the threat of losing it; we will never realise it's true value. Now that *"All About Eve: Your Women's Health Questions Answered"* is in your hands; you're a genius for taking control of your health and investing in it.

For anyone who has ever thought "I just can't ask ..." or "I'm afraid ..." or "What if..." — *"All About Eve: Your Women's Health Questions Answered"* is your doctor on-demand. A masterpiece of the best medical minds; 26 brilliant women doctors giving you easy to follow trusted advice on women's health. Their combined 17 areas of specialization will trace the stage of adulting where hair grows in places they are not supposed to, to losing hair in places where you don't want to.

This book gives readers the power to calm the overthinking chattering mind, the hope to turn illness into wellness and the strength to not give up.

Association of Women
Doctors (Singapore)

I don't know what tomorrow may bring or take away, but I know for sure that *"All about Eve: Your Women's Health Questions Answered"* will help me connect knowledge with action on my wellness journey.

The best gift you can give your family is a healthy you. I was just one of the very fortunate few that won the big lottery and got a second chance. Second chances are rare so if you have one chance in life — build your wealth in health.

Andrea De Cruz

CONTENTS

INTRODUCTION

Since its inception in 1998, the Association of Women Doctors Singapore (AWDS) has represented generations of Singapore female doctors and dentists. The association began as an ardent advocate and a voice for its members. Over time, its expertise has seen the association's role being expanded to benefit the wider community as well.

Over the years, AWDS has observed and keenly understands the myriad of responsibilities and roles of a modern woman. Daughter, mother, wife, caregiver, career woman, volunteer, advocate – it is common for many women to be juggling multiple roles at any given time. While being the key in maintaining healthy families, they often overlook their own physical, mental and even emotional health. This is made even more complicated because women live longer, experience unique health problems, and have higher rates of chronic health disease than men.

Through AWDS, we hope to inspire and motivate women to do more for their own health and well-being. We produce this book "**All about Eve: Your Women's Health Questions Answered**" during my tenure as President of the AWDS in 2018-2020. Within these pages, women can find comprehensive information about health issues they may have to navigate in every stage of life. This book is enabled by a generous "Seeds of Change" grant from Ministry of Social and Family Development and Singapore Council of Women's Organisations, staunch support from my executive committee members, as well as many hours of hard work by every member of my dream team consisting of my especially devoted co-editors Dr Annabel Chew and Dr Jade Kua, all authors and illustrators.

The book is divided into three parts and encompasses the entire journey from girlhood into womanhood.

The first part **"Overview of the female anatomy"** provides an overview of the changes the female body undergoes, from puberty to menopause.

"Stages of life and common problems at each stage" forms the second part of the book. The five sections within delve deeper into individual life stages and the common health problems that women may encounter.

In the ***Puberty*** section, we answer questions on what constitutes a normal menstrual cycle, how to support and guide adolescents, how to deal with eating disorders, and what are some common skin conditions associated with puberty.

Under the ***Young Womanhood*** section, we emphasise the choices women can make to empower themselves as they begin adulthood. We discuss the various methods of contraception, the importance of a PAP smear and the role of HPV vaccination in preventing cervical cancer.

In the section ***Starting a Family***, we explore issues on starting a family, the physiological changes in pregnancy and how to manage the physical and emotional changes that come with it, including anxiety and depression. Beyond that, we also debunk myths associated with breastfeeding, explain the causes of infertility and provide information on how to cope as a working mother.

In the section ***Middle-aged Women***, we dive into the common health conditions in this age group and how we should prevent, detect and live with them. These include breast and gynaecological cancers, diabetes and ischaemic heart disease.

We cover important topics of menopause, dementia under the section ***Mature Womanhood***, and provide information on the common but often neglected issues of aging including eye conditions, psychological health and how to achieve peace of mind by planning your legacy ahead for end of life.

"Bare essentials from cradle to grave" forms the third and final part of the book and looks at some salient health topics that are essential throughout one's lifetime. These include answers to the following questions: How do I get started on exercising? How do I develop and maintain good oral hygiene and dental health? What are the lifestyle changes that can help prevent depression and burnout? How do I improve the quality of my sex life and level of intimacy in my relationships?

Association of Women
Doctors (Singapore)

    This book is a project of ambition and heart. It consists of chapters written by dedicated women specialists in the topics they authored, in a clear and concise question and answer format, beautifully illustrated and comes with summary boxes outlining the key take home messages for every chapter.

    We hope that this book will reach out to women of all backgrounds, and empower them to become healthier and better versions of themselves. Because only when women understand how and why they should put their needs first, can our community continue to benefit from all that they selflessly give.

OVERVIEW OF THE FEMALE ANATOMY

Whilst the human body goes through many different changes throughout one's lifespan, the biggest anatomical differences that distinguish females from males happen during adolescence and menopause.

Puberty includes the biologic changes that adolescents encounter. On average, girls begin puberty between 8 to 11 years of age and their pubertal changes usually begin before boys of the same age. However being smaller or bigger than other girls is normal as each child experiences puberty at her own pace.

The first pubertal change is usually breast development, starting with a breast bud. At around age 9, a height spurt starts; and approximately one year after that, the menstrual periods begin. Pubic hair development happens usually shortly after breast development, but occasionally coincides with or even precedes breast development. By the time they are 12 years of age, most will have developed underarm hair.

During puberty, it is normal for the body shape to change. There may not only be an increase in height and weight, but the hips may get wider. There may also be an increase in fat in the buttocks, legs, and stomach. Adolescent girls might experience a sensation of clumsiness as their body size increases, with the feet, arms, legs, and hands initially growing faster. As the hormones

Dr Jade Kua is a Senior Consultant in General and Pediatric Emergency Medicine, and is also a professional life coach, and founder of Jade Life and Wellness.

of puberty increase, adolescents may experience an increase in oily skin and sweating. Acne may develop.

With physical changes in puberty, come mental and emotional changes that mark adolescence as well. Girls in these years begin to think abstractly and eventually make plans and set long-term goals. These tasks of adolescence include establishing an adult identity, seeking independence from adults, and establishing economic self-sufficiency; these tasks may begin before the teen years, and might not be completed until the early twenties.

The time that marks a young woman's life is usually between 18 to 35 years old, traditionally emphasised as her child-bearing years. Naturally, females are able to become pregnant once they have their first menstrual period; and increasingly, many women are able to bear children later on in life, with great leaps in medical techniques.

Perimenopause may begin several years before the last menstrual period. Signs of perimenopause include a disruption in frequency, regularity, length and volume of menstrual flow. Eventually a woman's periods will become much less frequent, until they stop completely for a year, and that is when menopause is established.

Menopause is a normal part of a woman's aging process. Most women experience menopause between 45 and 55 years old. During this time, the ovaries stop making the hormones oestrogen and progesterone, and stop releasing eggs. After menopause, a woman cannot become pregnant anymore.

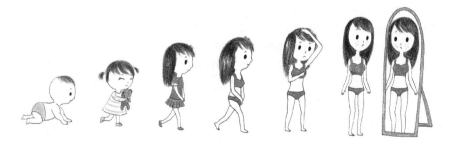

As hormone levels fall, vaginal walls become thinner, dryer, less elastic, and possibly more easily irritated, rendering sex painful and the risk of yeast infections higher. Women going through menopause experience hot flashes, moodiness, headaches, and trouble sleeping. They may notice in their bodies, a decrease in breast tissue and problems associated with bone loss. There may also be a loss of tone in the pubic muscles, resulting in the vagina, uterus or urinary bladder falling out of position (known as prolapse).

The term "older women" refers to women who have completed menopause, and the anatomical changes of ageing are related to loss of mass or function at a cellular or tissue level, reduced capacity of organ or system. With advanced age, older women may encounter loss of lean muscle mass, cardiovascular problems such as hypertension, depressed immune response, and fractures associated with loss of bone mass.

Any vaginal bleeding that occurs after menopause is abnormal and should be investigated. Older teaching focused on total removal of a woman's reproductive organs when disease sets in after the child-bearing years are over. Newer advances in technology focus on targeted removal of the disease itself, via infrared or high frequency ultrasound, allowing for preservation of one's femininity. This is an important concept that underpins treatment of older women, not just in Western medicine but in many traditional cultural practices too.

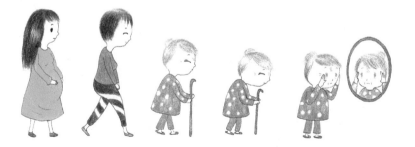

STAGES OF LIFE AND COMMON PROBLEMS AT EACH STAGE

PUBERTY

MENSTRUAL HEALTH

Take Home Points

1. Menstruation is a natural function that is an integral component of the reproductive health of women. If managed well, it can become a positive experience.

2. It is important to understand the physiological mechanism of normal menstrual function and what constituents a normal menstrual cycle.

3. Practice safe hygiene practices with regards to the menstrual cycle — such as changing pads/tampons frequently, and avoiding douching of the vagina.

4. Do recognise the challenges with menstruation and the coping mechanisms.

5. Do recognise potential problems associated with menses, and seek help early if there is abnormal vaginal discharge with or without abdominal pain and fever, absence of menses other than times mentioned, abnormal uterine bleeding with or without symptoms of anaemia like dizziness, chest pain, palpitations and breathlessness.

Dr Sonali Chonkar is a Senior Staff Physician in General Obstetrics and Gynaecology, and is currently practising at the KK Women's and Children's hospital. She is also an Adjunct Assistant Professor at Duke-NUS Medical School and Yong Loo Lin School of Medicine.

What is menstruation and what constitutes a normal menstrual cycle?

Menstruation is a natural function that allows the lining of the womb (uterus) to be shed in the form of blood from the vagina every month and is an essential component for the reproductive health of women and adolescent girls. Menstruation is also sometimes known as 'menses' or as a 'menstrual period'.

Components of a normal menstrual cycle include cycle frequency, duration, volume and regularity. The parameters of a 'normal' menstrual cycle are adapted from Munro *et al.*, 2018 as below.[1]

A normal menstrual cycle length is the number of days from the first day of bleeding in one menstrual cycle to the first day of bleeding in the next with no more than between 7–9 days of difference between the shortest to longest cycles.

Normal frequency of menses (days) is about 24–38 days.

Normal duration, that is number of days bleeding in a single menstrual period is ≤ 8 days.

Normal volume of menstrual blood loss is anything that does not interfere with a woman's physical, social, emotional, and/or quality of life.

When does menstruation start and end?

Menstruation usually starts at menarche which is typically between the ages of 10 and 19 years of age, alongside development of physical changes (e.g., breast and body hair development, widening of hips, amongst others) and emotional changes. It normally ceases at menopause, usually around the late forties.

There are times when there may be absence of periods (amenorrhea) or irregular periods such as:

- Breastfeeding — This usually delays the return of normal menstruation postpartum, particularly if exclusive and may form the basis for the lactation amenorrhoea method (LAM) of contraception for the first six months of the baby's life
- Rapid weight change — increase or decrease
- Body weight below a certain level — e.g., due to eating disorders such as anorexia nervosa
- Emotional stress

- Excess physical stress
- Significant illness
- Medication — e.g., hormones, cytotoxics, some psychotropic drugs (e.g., risperidone)
- Pregnancy
- At the time of menarche (when menstruation first begins) and following menopause when menstruation ceases.

Experience of amenorrhea or irregular periods may need assessment and appropriate management wherever deemed necessary.

What is the physiological mechanism involved?

Following menstruation, the lining of the uterus begins to develop under the influence of hormones to prepare the uterus for receiving a fertilised egg. Around day 14 of each cycle, an egg is released from one of the ovaries (ovulation) and moves through the fallopian tubes into the uterus. If the egg is not fertilised, the lining of the uterus then detaches and is shed through the vagina along with blood as menses. The process repeats itself throughout the reproductive phase of the woman from menarche to menopause.

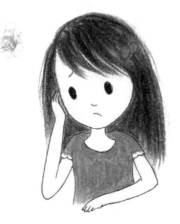

What can I expect during a menstrual period?

It is normal to experience cramps or lower abdominal pain, nausea, headaches, tiredness, feeling faint, lower back pain and general discomfort like bloating and breast tenderness which may begin a few days before the onset of blood loss (pre-menstrual symptoms). It is also common to experience emotional changes such as feelings of sadness, irritability or anger and these are due to fluctuations in hormones. The symptoms widely vary from woman to woman and can be managed on individual basis. Pain during periods (dysmenorrhea) often has no underlying medical explanation and studies report varying prevalence.

Will I be at any risk due to menstruation?

Menstruation is a natural, healthy process, but if not properly managed, may result in health problems which can be compounded by social, cultural and religious practices.

There may be potential risks that result from poor menstrual hygiene management. These include:

Health risks from sanitary products

There may be hypersensitivity reactions in some women with sensitive skin, particularly as a result of friction or prolonged contact of moisture with the skin. Some may experience allergic reactions to additives such as those used to mask odour and/or increase absorbency. However, most manufacturers ensure that their products are rigorously tested for quality and sold under hygienic conditions.

Toxic shock syndrome

This is a rare but dangerous syndrome caused by a toxin produced by the bacterium, Staphylococcus aureus and can be fatal in a small percentage (5 percent) of cases. This bacteria is common on the skin and in mucous membranes such as the lining of the nose and mouth. It usually follows skin irritation or infection, and is usually linked to the use of tampons and intravaginal contraceptive devices.

The risk of infection is higher than normal during menstruation because the cervix is usually open to allow blood to pass out. Theoretically this can predispose entry of bacteria into the uterus. This is further aided by change in the pH of the vagina which becomes less acidic at this time, making yeast infections more likely. Certain practices are more likely to increase the risk of infection. These include prolonged use of the same pad for extended periods of time, douching of vagina (inserting liquid into the vagina), wiping from back to front following defecation or urination which allows harmful bacteria, such as *Escherichia coli* (*E. coli*) from the anus to contaminate the genital tract that could lead to infection. These additional risks mean that ensuring good hygiene during menstruation is very important.

How do I know that I have an infection?

There may be appearance of abnormal discharge indicating onset of infection. Normal vaginal discharge is thin and clear, thick and mucous-like, or long and stringy depending on the time in menstrual cycle. Discharge that indicates a health problem may be accompanied by itching, rash or soreness. It may be persistent, profuse, and/or lumpy like cottage cheese. It may be grey/white or yellow/green with a foul smell. It may complicate to cause lower abdominal pain and fever. If untreated it can have implications such as blocked fallopian tubes and pelvic abscesses which may adversely affect future fertility and increase the risk of ectopic pregnancy.

What are some challenges that women encounter due to menstruation and its impact?

Generation gaps lead to different opinions and attitudes towards menstruation. Conservative mothers from the older generation tend to believe that the use of tampons could tear a female's hymen thereby causing them to lose their virginity.[2]

Gender based biases cause males to be less considerate, less empathetic and not willing to openly discuss issues related to menses or having open conversations in general.

The social stigma of menstruation forces young women going through their periods to feel ashamed or embarrassed. When women encounter difficult and uncomfortable situations, they often choose to conceal and keep mum about their discomfort, instead of seeking help or advice from their peers, particularly male friends and/or family members. Lack of open dialogue to discuss issues surrounding menstruation predisposes women to experience psycho-social stress and possibly dismiss serious issues related to their menstrual health, such as endometriosis, which could affect fertility[3] and cause them to suffer from chronic pelvic pain.

Women who are going through menstruation at work often do not feel that they can talk to others, particularly men, for the things they need, be it a sanitary pad or a sick day. This is due to a common male belief that when women have their 'period', it makes them weak, moody or even unreliable.[4] According to the American Academy of Family Physicians, up to 20 percent of women suffer from menstrual cramping severe enough to interfere with daily activities. But many menstruating women would rather tolerate their pain and suffer in silence instead of seeking help.[5] Many women may also choose to miss hours or even entire days of work just to avoid having to manage their menstruation in distressing environments.[6] Thus, this in turn could result in lower productivity levels in the workplace.

How can I overcome these challenges?

Sharing menstrual experiences with others:

1. Encourage open conversations between both genders
2. Encourage and equip parents to have positive discussions about menstruation from young
3. Talk to other girls and women, such as your mother, sister, aunt, grandmother, or female friends.

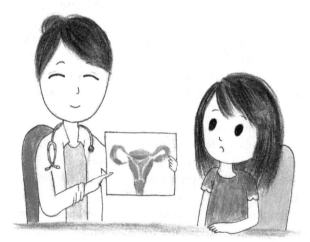

When should I seek help?

When you experience abnormal uterine bleeding (AUB) and pain

Abnormal uterine bleeding is any variation from the parameters of a normal menstrual cycle. It is a broad term that encompasses several forms of menstrual dysfunction as below:

- Heavy bleeding during the period (HMB)
- Bleeding or spotting between periods
- Bleeding or spotting after sex
- Menstrual cycles that are longer than 38 days or shorter than 24 days
- Prolonged periods in which bleeding lasts more than 7–9 days.

Heavy menstrual bleeding (HMB)

It is excessive menstrual blood loss (MBL) that interferes with the physical, social, emotional and/or material quality of life.

AUB and its sub-group, heavy menstrual bleeding (HMB) affects around 14 to 25 percent of women of reproductive age.

About 1 in 20 women aged between 30–49 years of age consult their GPs each year because of heavy periods or menstrual problems. HMB is the most common condition seen in both primary as well as secondary care settings and, along with other menstrual disorders, comprise 12 percent of all gynaecological referrals. Some of the causes of abnormal bleeding include the following:

- Problems with ovulation
- Fibroids and polyps
- A condition in which the endometrium grows into the wall of the uterus (Adenomyosis).
- Bleeding disorders
- Problems linked to some birth control methods, such as an intrauterine device (IUD) or birth control pills
- Miscarriage
- Ectopic pregnancy
- Certain types of cancer, such as cancer of the uterus.

Chronic pelvic pain

Chronic pelvic pain in women is defined as persistent, non-cyclic pain perceived to be in structures related to the pelvis. An arbitrary duration of

6 months is usually considered chronic. There is often no specific etiological factor and it is usually associated with other functional somatic pain syndromes (e.g., irritable bowel syndrome, non-specific chronic fatigue syndrome) and mental health disorders (e.g., post-traumatic stress disorder, depression).

Some of the causes of pelvic pain include the following:

- Adenomyosis, endometriosis
- Fibroids
- Adhesions
- Certain types of cancer, such as cancer of the endometrium, ovary
- Interstitial cystitis, urethral syndrome
- Inflammatory bowel disease, irritable bowel syndrome
- Musculoskeletal etiologies
- Nerve entrapment
- Mental health issues.

References

1. Munro MG, Critchley HO, and Fraser IS (2018), The two FIGO systems for normal and abnormal uterine bleeding symptoms and classification of causes of abnormal uterine bleeding in the reproductive years: 2018 revisions. *Int J Gynecol Obstet*, 143: 393–408. https://doi.org/10.1002/ijgo.12666
2. AFP. (2020, March 02). Talking about a menstrual revolution: Asia's period problems. Retrieved November 05, 2020, from https://www.asiaone.com/lifestyle/talking-about-menstrual-revolution-asias-period-problems
3. United Nations. (n.d.). Break taboo around menstruation, act to end 'disempowering discrimination, say UN experts | | UN news. United Nations. Retrieved November 4, 2021, from https://news.un.org/en/story/2019/03/1034131#:~:text=%E2%80%9CStigma%20around%20.
4. Berwick, I. (2019, October 17). Why the stigma of periods is open for discussion. Retrieved from https://www.ft.com/content/374d6702-d0ba-11e9-b018-ca4456540ea6
5. Aufrichtig, A. (2016, October 24). Period pain: Why do so many women suffer from Menstrual Cramps in silence? *The Guardian*. Retrieved November 4, 2021, from https://www.theguardian.com/lifeandstyle/2016/oct/24/period-pain-menstruation-cramps-dysmenorrhea

6. Sommer M, Chandraratna S, Cavill S, Mahon T and Phillips-Howard P. (2016). Managing menstruation in the workplace: an overlooked issue in low- and middle-income countries. *International Journal for Equity in Health*, 15(1): 1–5.

Further Reading

Chronic pelvic pain — what you should know. *Am Fam Physician* 2008; 77(11):1544. Available at: https://www.aafp.org/afp/2008/0601/p1544. html;Chronic Pelvic Pain. Familydoctor.org; 2019, Nov 7. Available at: https://familydoctor.org/familydoctor/en/diseases-conditions/chronic-pelvic-pain.html.

Haver J and Long J. Menstrual hygiene management — operational guidelines. Savethechildren.org. Available at: https://www.savethechildren.org/content/dam/global/reports/health-and-nutrition/mens-hyg-mgmt-guide.pdf

Haver J and Long JL. (2015). Menstrual Hygiene Management Operational Guideline. Retrieved from https://resourcecentre.savethechildren.net/pdf/menstrual_hygiene_management_operational_guidelines.pdf/

Heavy menstrual bleeding: Assessment and management: Guidance. Heavy menstrual bleeding: assessment and management. (2018, March 14). Retrieved November 4, 2021, from https://www.nice.org.uk/guidance/ng88.

Heavy menstrual bleeding. costing report — implementing NICE guidance in England. National Institute for Health and Clinical Excellence; 2007, Jan. Available at: https://elearning.rcog.org.uk/sites/default/files/Abnormal%20 uterine%20bleeding/NICE_HMB_costing_CG44_2007.pdf

Menstruation. MedlinePlus; 2020, Jun 15. Available at: https://medlineplus. gov/menstruation.html#:~:text=Menstruation%2C%20or%20 period%2C%20is%20normal,tissue%20from%20inside%20the%20uterus

Ortiz DD. (n.d.). Chronic pelvic pain in women — AAFP home . Retrieved November 4, 2021, from https://www.aafp.org/afp/2008/0601/ afp20080601p1535.pdf.

U.S. National Library of Medicine. (2021, October 18). Menstruation | period. *MedlinePlus*. Retrieved November 4, 2021, from https://medlineplus.gov/menstruation.html.

ADOLESCENT HEALTH: PSYCHOSOCIAL EFFECTS OF PUBERTY

Take Home Points

1. Adolescence is a period of rapid physical, psychological and cognitive growth that lasts from ages 10 to 19. This period of maturation is not complete until the end of young adulthood at approximately 24 years of age.
2. Due to the tempo of adolescent brain development, adolescents may be vulnerable to participating in risk taking behaviour as they may overvalue rewards and undervalue the consequences of behaviour.
3. Adolescents benefit from ongoing guidance, involvement, and support from adults, including parents, guardians, family members, and teachers.
4. Proper sleep, nutrition, and physical activity is important for adolescents' physical and mental health.

(Continued)

Dr Courtney Davis is a Senior Staff Physician in Adolescent medicine service, and is currently practising at the KK Women's and Children's hospital.

(*Continued*)

> 5. Parents and guardians should communicate with their adolescents regarding sensitive topics such as sex, tobacco and substance use because parents and guardians are important and influential sources of information for adolescents.

What is adolescence?

Adolescence is a phase of growth and change that spans from the ages of 10 to 19 years. An adolescent experiences rapid physical, psychological, and cognitive growth. This period of maturation continues until the end of young adulthood at approximately 24 years of age.[1]

What are the physical changes that happen during adolescence and why is it important?

The physical changes associated with adolescence are the most visible and usually start in early adolescence (ages 9 to 14). For girls, they include rapid growth in height and weight, the development of breasts and hips and the start of menstruation. Adolescent females also experience an increase in body hair, perspiration, and oil production in skin and hair. This is also a period for muscle growth and accretion of bone density.[2] Thus, healthy eating habits are important to support this period of rapid growth and development and to achieve full growth potential as adults.

Why do adolescents behave so differently from children and adults?

Goals and tasks of adolescents differ from that of childhood and adulthood. Tasks of adolescents include achieving the goal of independence, forming self-identity and developing healthy peer relationships and body image.[1]

Adolescents start to think differently and begin to have an increased capacity for abstract and complex thought. They also develop a growing ability to set goals and work towards them.[1]

The hallmark of adolescence is a growing sense of self-identity and increased independence. Adolescents are more likely to test boundaries and rules, and some adolescents may have increased conflicts with their family members. As they continue to mature during this stage, they develop a firmer sense of self-identity, increased emotional stability, increased concern for others and improved self-reliance. Their relationships with peers become stronger and some may start to have more serious romantic relationships.[1]

Given the physical changes, influence of social media and increased awareness of peers, these young people may feel conscious and awkward about themselves and their bodies. They may also have increased mood swings.

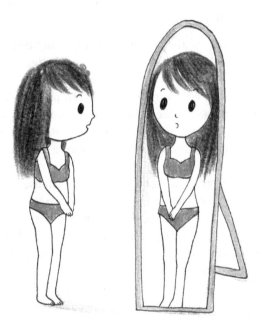

What happens to the brain during adolescence and does that affect behaviour?

Puberty initiates processes which lead to structural remodeling of the teenage brain. Apart from early childhood (ages 0–3), early adolescence (ages 9–14) is the other period in which rapid growth and development occur in the brain.[1]

During adolescence, the amygdala (which controls passion, impulse, fear, and aggression) develops faster than the part of the brain (the prefrontal cortex) that is responsible for planning and reasoning.

The prefrontal cortex is not fully developed until age 25. Thus, adolescents are more likely to engage in risk-taking behaviour, and over-value rewards without sufficient consideration of long-term consequences.

Furthermore, due to the timing of the maturation of other parts of the brain, adolescents are naturally more motivated by rewards than consequences, which may result in poor decision making.

How can I support my adolescent through this period and when should I start preparing?

Given the changes in the brain's development, teens are uniquely vulnerable to risk-seeking behaviours and supportive adults, including parents, play an important role to reduce this risk.

Starting early is the best way for parents to prepare for their child's adolescence. Providing a safe, supportive home environment, and developing a healthy parent-child relationship with open and respectful communication during childhood, is important for a smoother transition to adolescence.[1]

Adolescents need guidance and support to choose healthy ways of expressing their emerging self-identity (new hairstyle, new co-curricular activity, performing new talents in front of an audience) and guided away from dangerous risks (experimentation with alcohol and cigarettes, risky sexual behaviour). Thus, investing in, supporting, and mentoring adolescents is critical to get them and keep them on the right track.

Physical Health

What are healthy eating habits for a teenager?

Healthy eating habits formed in adolescence can form an important foundation for future adult health. Teens need appropriate eating habits to provide sufficient nutrition for this rapid period of growth. They should eat regular meals and snacks including sufficient proteins, fats and carbohydrates in accordance with the Health Promotion Board's My Healthy Plate guidelines. They should aim to eat 2 servings of fruits and 2 servings of vegetables each day. They should try to eat a variety of fruits and vegetables. Teenage females need sufficient vitamin D and calcium to ensure optimal bone health. They should aim for at least two cups of milk a day or calcium-fortified milk alternatives.[3] Eating meals as a family also benefits both their physical and mental health.

What are warning signs that my teen is not eating well?

For any growth concerns, please see your family physician or general practitioner (GP). Both height and weight increase rapidly during adolescence and growth should follow a similar pattern as the pre-pubertal period. Weight loss, lack of weight gain, or excessive weight gain out of proportion to height gain may be abnormal in adolescence and should be evaluated by your family physician or GP. Skipping meals, dieting, or significant changes in types or portions of food being consumed should be evaluated by a physician. These changes in eating habits or weight loss can be a warning sign for an eating disorder (see Chapter 3.1.3).

What are the benefits of physical activity?

Teens need appropriate opportunities for exercise and movement. Regular physical activity has significant health benefits for teenagers, including improved aerobic fitness, body composition and musculoskeletal health, as well as decreased risk of metabolic disease. Moreover, regular physical activity improves adolescent mental health, academic performance, and sleep.[4]

Singapore's Integrated 24-hour Movement Guidelines recommend that children and adolescents should participate in a daily average of 60 minutes of moderate to vigorous physical activity and engage in muscle and bone strengthening exercises 3 times a week. They should also incorporate light physical activity and movement breaks into their day. It is important to note that adolescents should take necessary precautions before, during and after exercise and see a physician if they feel unwell during exercise.[4]

Why is sleep important and how much should my teen sleep?

Sufficient sleep is critical for teens' physical and mental health.[5] Teens should obtain appropriate amounts of sleep during adolescence. Current guidelines recommend at least 9 hours of sleep a night for ages 7–13, 8 hours of sleep a night for ages 14–17 and 7 hours of sleep a night for those older than 18 years of age.[4,5]

What should my teen do if he/she is unable to sleep?

After puberty, there is a shift in a teenager's internal clock, meaning that a teenager tends to fall asleep later and also wake up later in the morning. Thus, it is important to instil good sleep hygiene as a routine. Teens should try to sleep and wake up at a similar time each day and avoid oversleeping on the weekend. Limiting the use of digital devices prior to bedtime can aid in proper sleep, as the light from the devices can stimulate the brain and prolong wakefulness. It is also helpful to avoid caffeinated drinks. Establishing sleep and bedtime routines such as reading a book before bed or taking a shower can signal to the body that it is time to sleep. Getting sufficient exercise and sunlight during the daytime can also be beneficial. If teens have persistent difficulties sleeping or are awakening at night frequently, they should see a GP to evaluate any physical and emotional health concerns that may be contributing to their poor sleeping habits.[5,6]

How will seeing the doctor be different once my child is an adolescent?

As adolescence is a transition to adulthood, this is an important time for them to start playing a more active role in their health. When parents and physicians feel the adolescent is ready, he/she should assume greater responsibility for taking his/her medications. The adolescent should start to know the names of medications that he/she takes regularly, and the timings and dosages. Of course, for some adolescents or for adolescents with certain medical conditions, parental supervision may still be important. The adolescent's physician may start to spend part of their clinic consult speaking to the adolescent without the parent being present so as to build their independence.

Sexual Health

What changes in sexuality occur in adolescence?

During adolescence, it is common that youth may start to explore their sexuality and sexual identity. This may include the development of sexual or romantic feelings, exploring their sexual identity, and, for some adolescents, the initiation of some forms of sexual activity or physical affection.

Why should parents talk to their adolescents about sex and sexuality?

While adolescents receive many messages regarding sexual identity and activity from peers and the media, parents play a critical role in helping them to develop healthy mindsets regarding sexuality and sexual identity, as well as influence responsible decision-making about sexual activity. One key message to highlight is that no one has the right to pressure them to have sex or engage in other sexual activities that make them uncomfortable.[7]

While these topics may be uncomfortable to talk about with an adolescent, it is important to have open communication with teens and be able to provide them with reliable information regarding protecting themselves from sexually transmitted infections and pregnancy.[7] Teenagers whose parents talk to them about sex are more likely to put off having sex until they are older. They are also more likely to use contraceptives when they engage in sex.

It is never too early to talk to your child about their bodies and puberty. Experts recommend using the correct names for private body parts in these discussions. There are age-appropriate resources to guide these conversations.[8,9]

What should adolescents know about healthy romantic relationships?

Adolescents may start to form romantic relationships during this period of development. It is important for them to recognize signs of healthy relationships, including: respect for one another, settling disagreements peacefully, having common interests but also maintaining independent activities and friends outside of the relationship.[10]

Warning signs of an unhealthy relationship include a lack of respect, controlling behaviour, getting blamed for a partner's problems, behaviour which is overly jealous, controlling or possessive, or any form of verbal, physical, or sexual abuse.[10]

Emotional and Mental Health

How can I keep my adolescent emotionally healthy?

Parents, extended family, friends, caring adults, and teachers all play a critical role in supporting teens' emotional health. Some ways that parents or other trusted adults can help to promote adolescent mental health include: showing an interest in the adolescents' lives, spending time with them individually and as a family, and helping them to develop problem-solving skills.[11]

It is important to help adolescents develop self-esteem by showing love, affection and care for them. This includes praising their efforts as well as accomplishments, showing interest in their activities, and helping them to learn to set realistic goals and means of achieving them. Trusted adults can help by listening, respecting their feelings, and having open communication with their teen(s).[11]

Parents play an important role in creating a positive and safe home environment. Sufficient sleep, regular meals, and physical activity are important for mental health. Moreover, parents should be aware of the adolescent's media use with regards to content, amount of time spent, and who they are interacting with online.[11]

How can I help build my adolescent's emotional resilience?

It is important to help youth learn how to problem-solve. One way to do this is to talk over solutions and ideas with them, without taking over. Encourage them to deal with problems and feelings as they arise, rather than let the issues build up. It is helpful to teach them skills to help them relax when needed, such as calming activities, deep breathing, time alone, and exercise. Adolescents should be encouraged to talk to trusted family members, friends, teachers, or school counsellors.[11]

What are some warning signs that an adolescent may need help?

Adolescents may show different warning signs that they need help. If parents or loved ones are concerned about an adolescent's mental health, it is good to seek help from trusted professionals such as school teachers or counselor, mental health professional, or a GP. It is advisable to seek help early.

Some warning signs may include an adolescent appearing down or sad all the time, feeling hopeless or lacking interest, or exhibiting aggressive or disobedient behaviour. Other warning signs include persistent worries or fears, difficulty managing everyday activities, sudden behaviour changes, and decline in school attendance or performance. Having problems getting along with friends and avoiding social activities, can also indicate signs of difficulty in managing peer relations. Physical complaints such as headaches, stomach aches, and sleep difficulties can also be warning signs.[11] Chapter 4.3 discusses mental wellness in greater detail.

How should an adolescent get help if required?

If you suspect that an adolescent may require help for his/her physical, emotional or mental health, it is good to discuss your concerns with an appropriate professional such as a school teacher, school counsellor, physician, social worker or mental health professional. It is helpful to express concern and care for the adolescent and to take his/her concerns seriously.

Digital Health

Why is my teenager 'online' so much?

Adolescents engage in a range of activities online. They may be using the internet as a tool for studying, or to learn more about their interests. They may also be using the internet to connect with others through social media, engage in online games, create or find interesting digital media, and join interest groups. In doing so, they may cultivate virtual relationships with individuals they know in person, or purely on an online basis.[12]

How much screen time should my adolescent have?

Teens should try to limit recreational screen time to no more than two hours a day.[4]

What are the benefits to using online technology for teens?

Adolescents can access information to educate themselves. They can use technology to make and maintain friendships, and cultivate a sense of belonging through staying connected. Technology can also aid in identify formation — through learning and talking.[12]

How can I guide my teenager in the use of technology?

While technology can have many benefits for teens, it can also have risks. It is important for parents or caregivers to be involved in negotiating boundaries for technology, including media type, amounts of screen time, and online behaviours. It is also important for parents to review digital safety with their adolescents and have an awareness of their adolescent's online activities.[12]

Risks of technology use include cyberbullying, that is, using technology to bully someone, and trolling where people intentionally attempt to upset others on the internet and cause considerable distress. Isolation may occur when too much time is spent online, at the expense of face-to-face time with friends and family. Adolescents may post inappropriate pictures or content online which may end up causing problems or embarrassment for themselves or others. Finally, there is a risk that teens may form inappropriate relationships with strangers online, that may be detrimental to their health and safety.[12]

While it may be best to avoid real life meetups, with new friends that they have met online, teens may still choose to do so. Parents should encourage their adolescents to inform them prior to meeting with any new online acquaintances. Parents and adolescents must remember that online acquaintances may not be truthful about their age, or very different from who they portray themselves to be online. In these situations, teens must exercise extreme caution when meeting these acquaintances. Safety measures should include meeting in a well-populated public place and having someone accompanying them to the meetup.

What are warning signs of digital addiction for adolescents?

There are many signs of digital addiction for adolescents. These include increased time spent on digital devices, becoming depressed or irritable without a device, spending less time with family and friends, deteriorating eating and sleep patterns, as well as personal hygiene, and declining school attendance and academic performance. If you are worried about your adolescent, it is good to seek help or a professional assessment.[13]

Substance Use

Adolescents may experiment with or initiate regular use of substances such as tobacco, alcohol, vaping, and recreational drugs. This experimentation may be partially due to the brain changes that cause adolescents to undervalue consequences. Use of tobacco, alcohol, vape, and recreational drugs can have significant health (short and long term) and legal consequences for adolescents.[14]

It is important to start talking about the risks of smoking and substance use in a developmentally appropriate fashion with children when they are still young.

Parents are important role models and open parental communication can reduce adolescent smoking. While parents are encouraged to provide adolescents with an appropriate amount of freedom, it is important to set firm family guidelines on acceptable and unacceptable behaviour, including regarding substance use. However, if your adolescent is already smoking, try to engage in open communication, find out why he/she is smoking, and how to encourage him/her to quit. Similar to adults, it can be challenging for young people to stop smoking and they will benefit from encouragement and support.[14]

If your child is having an issue with tobacco or any other substance, seek guidance from a healthcare professional for further assessment and treatment options.

References

1. Sawyer S, Afifi R, Bearinger L, Blakemore S, Dick B, Ezeh A, *et al.* Adolescence: a foundation for future health. *Lancet* 2012; 379(9826):1630–1640. Available at: https://pubmed.ncbi.nlm.nih. gov/22538178/.
2. Wood C, Lane L, Cheetham T. Puberty: Normal physiology (brief overview). *Best Pract Res Clinical Endocrino Metab* 2019 Jun; 33(3). Available at: https://pubmed.ncbi.nlm.nih.gov/31000487/.
3. Healthy Food for Kids and Teens. Health Hub; 2021 Aug 19. Available at: https://www.healthhub.sg/live-healthy/578/A%20Healthy%20 Food%20Foundation%20-%20for%20Kids%20and%20Teens.
4. Academy of Medicine Singapore College of Paediatrics and Child Health Singapore. Consensus Statement: Singapore Integrated 24-hour Movement Guidelines for Children and Adolescents. Singapore; 2021 Jan.
5. Owens J. Insufficient sleep in adolescents and young adults: an update on causes and consequences. *Pediatrics* 2014; 134(3): e921–932. Available at: https://pediatrics.aappublications.org/content/134/3/e921.
6. SingHealth DukeNUS Sleep Centre. What do we know about sleep in adolescence? SingHealth Medical News; 2018 Mar. Available at: https:// www.singhealth.com.sg/news/medical-news/sleep-in-adolescence.
7. Adolescent Sexuality: Talk the Talk Before They Walk the Walk. Healthy Children; 2009 Feb. Available at: https://healthychildren.org/English/ ages-stages/teen/dating-sex/Pages/Adolescent-Sexuality-Talk-the-Talk-Before-They-Walk-the-Walk.aspx.
8. Ashcraft AM, Murray PJ. Talking to parents about adolescent sexuality. *Pediatr Clin North Am* 2017 Apr; 64(2): 305–320. doi: 10.1016/ j.pcl.2016.11.002.

9. How to Talk to Your Kids About Sex. Health Hub; 2021 Sep. Available at: https://www.healthhub.sg/live-healthy/960/how-to-talk-to-your-kids-about-sex.

10. Expect Respect: Healthy Relationships. Healthy Children; 2009 Feb. Available at: https://www.healthychildren.org/English/ages-stages/teen/dating-sex/Pages/Expect-Respect-Healthy-Relationships.aspx

11. Teen Mental Health: Supporting your Child. Raising Children Network; 2021 May. Available at: https://raisingchildren.net.au/pre-teens/mental-health-physical-health/about-mental-health/teen-mental-health.

12. Technology and Teenagers. Reach Out; 2021. Available at: https://parents.au.reachout.com/skills-to-build/wellbeing/technology-and-teenagers.

13. Signs & Symptoms. National Addictions Management Service (NAMS). Available at: https://www.nams.sg/helpseekers/internet-and-gaming/Pages/Signs%20and%20Symptoms.aspx.

14. Have a Minute? Talk to Your Kids about Smoking. Health Hub; 2021 Jun. Available from: https://www.healthhub.sg/live-healthy/909/have-a-minute-talk-to-your-kids-about-smoking.

EATING DISORDERS

Take Home Points

1. Eating disorders are serious psychiatric illnesses that can result in physiological complications.
2. The types of eating disorders are: Anorexia Nervosa, Bulimia Nervosa, Binge Eating Disorder, Avoidant Restrictive Food Intake Disorder, Other Specified Eating/Feeding Disorders, Unspecified Eating/Feeding Disorders.
3. Individuals with eating disorders often present with other comorbid conditions such as depression, anxiety etc.
4. Some individuals may be more prone to developing eating disorders, however, there are preventive measures that can be employed.
5. Eating disorders are treatable, and recovery is possible — psychiatric, psychological and nutritional management is available, as well as other forms of therapies such as art therapy and family therapy.

Dr Ng Kah Wee is a Senior Consultant Psychiatrist, and Head of the Eating Disorders Program, specializing in Eating Disorders and General Psychiatry, and is currently practising at the Singapore General Hospital.

Dr Kim Lian Rolles-Abraham is a Senior Clinical Psychologist and Head of Therapy Services, specializing in Eating Disorders and General Psychology, and is currently practising at Better Life Psychological Medicine Clinic.

What are eating disorders?

Eating disorders constitute a category of major psychiatric conditions and this group of disorders is rather unique because they are often associated with medical morbidity such as acute electrolyte abnormalities, blood pressure changes, chronic effects such as bone mineral density changes, renal scarring, gastritis and constipation. It is also closely associated with secondary co-morbid psychiatric symptoms like depression, anxiety, self-harm behaviours and even suicide. Patients with eating disorders may have body image preoccupation or distortion, experience intense fear of weight gain and may develop behaviours of starvation, binge-eating and self-induced vomiting. Often, such behaviours impact one's socio-occupational function and well-being, which is one of the main features of a psychiatric disorder. Broadly speaking, we can categorise eating disorders into the following: Anorexia Nervosa; Bulimia Nervosa; Binge Eating Disorder; Avoidant Restrictive Food Intake Disorder; Other Specified Feeding / Eating Disorders; Unspecified Feeding/Eating Disorders.

A) *Anorexia Nervosa*

This type of eating disorder is typically characterised by behaviours such as restrictive eating, dieting practices, excessive exercise and even binge-eating and self-induced vomiting, resulting in a significant loss of weight and becoming underweight as a result. There is usually prominent fear of weight gain and body image concerns surrounding body size and shape. In some patients, menstruation might have stopped completely for months because of the significant starvation. Patients in this category are usually of a younger age at presentation, namely, in their pubescent years or late teens.

B) *Bulimia Nervosa*

Bulimia Nervosa is rather similar to the aforementioned category, with the discerning characteristic that patients diagnosed with this condition are usually of normal weight. They should also have regular patterns of binge-eating episodes with behaviours of compensation such as self-induced vomiting, use of laxatives or diuretics, starvation or excessive exercise.

Usually, patients in this category present at a slightly later age, perhaps in the late teens or early to mid-twenties.

C) *Binge Eating Disorder*

This condition is now a diagnosis of its own in the Diagnostic and Statistical Manual of Mental Disorders (DSM-5) and it is characterised by regular binge-eating episodes but without compensatory behaviours. Patients who fall into this category are usually males, present at a later age and might have developed chronic medical conditions such as dyslipidaemia or Type II diabetes mellitus by the time they seek help for mental health issues.

D) *Avoidant Restrictive Food Intake/Feeding Disorder*

This condition is gaining recognition since it was introduced in the DSM-5, updated in 2013. It generally describes a form of eating disorder which begins with a restricted intake from a very young age, not driven by intention to lose weight nor body image concerns. The restriction of intake may often be associated with other features such as consistency or colour or the taste of a certain food. Such restrictive eating would have resulted in significant weight loss and possibly stunting of growth since symptoms would have started at a young age.

E) *Other Specified Feeding/Eating Disorders*

Previously known as Eating Disorders — Not Otherwise Specified (EDNOS) in the previous DSM-4, this category of eating disorders include disorders which do not fulfil that of the preceding diagnoses. Generally, diagnoses we see in this category would include Atypical Anorexia Nervosa, Subthreshold Bulimia Nervosa and Night Eating syndrome.

F) *Unspecified Feeding/Eating Disorders*

This category would describe the rest of the eating disorders which do not have any specific patterns of behaviours which would allow them to be classified under the aforementioned diagnoses, but which still result in significant distress or psychosocial dysfunction.

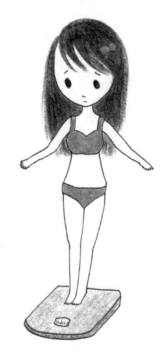

Am I at risk of getting an eating disorder?

As with most psychiatric conditions, there are usually multiple causative factors resulting in the development of the disorder. Biologically, one who has a relative or a close family member with an eating disorder is at a higher risk of developing one. Families which tend to body shame, be critical of one another, or have highly enmeshed intra-familial ties sometimes predispose their family members to developing an eating disorder. Sometimes we see patients develop an eating disorder after having lost significant amounts of weight from a physical illness — the weight loss and concerns with body image persists even after resolution of the bout of physical illness. Sometimes certain medications might have caused a sudden weight gain and inadvertently triggered the onset of an eating disorder. Steroids, certain selected antidepressants and antipsychotics, and thyroid medication are some examples.

Certain psychosocial stressors are also common features associated with the onset of an eating disorder. Going through phases of puberty, struggles with gender identity, being victims of domestic violence or sexual abuse are some of the associations we might notice in patients with eating disorders. Going through certain stages in life may also predispose a person to development of an eating disorder, for example, transition from the various levels of schooling (i.e., from primary to secondary school), marital discord, separation and divorce between parents, adjustment from having to live overseas, peri-partum periods wherein weight gain might have been significant. Having a concurrent struggle with another psychiatric disorder, for example depression, anxiety or obsessive compulsive disorder can be possible precipitating factors for the development of an eating disorder. It has also been thought that certain personalities types tend to suffer from a certain type of eating disorder. The more widely known being that people who are perfectionistic in nature tend to develop the restrictive type of eating disorder whilst people with more chaotic predispositions and lifestyles tend to have more binge and purge patterns of behaviours.

So, in summary, one can possibly develop a eating disorder at any stage of life, though we do know Anorexia Nervosa tends to strike particularly during the early teens and pubertal years, whilst Bulimia Nervosa tends to have its onset in the later teens and early twenties. However, we have come across patients who might have developed an eating disorder at other stages of life and age groups, secondary to the various stressors mentioned above.

How can I prevent it?

Maintaining a healthy relationship with food and exercise, taking care to not be overly excessive on either as a coping mechanism will be a good start. Anecdotally, some of our patients started off with a coping strategy of comfort eating or exercising, but this got out of hand and spiralled into a full-blown eating disorder. Maintaining one's mental health and ensuring any existing psychiatric condition is well controlled will also be key. Keeping to a regular sleep — wake cycle and having a well varied number of coping skills are definitely good ways to keep eating disorders at bay. This is especially true given the current COVID pandemic, when usual destressing methods such as meeting friends over a meal, playing sports together or engaging in recreational exercise can be very suddenly restricted because of the necessary social distancing measures put in place.

Keeping the channels of communication open and accessible between family members is also very important. Most people do rely on our families and next of kin to help with our problems. On the flipside, sometimes tensions from lack of communication and strained family ties might have triggered the onset of the disorder. Having a supportive parent, spouse or significant other has definitely proved to be a positive factor in each of our patients' prognosis and recovery journey.

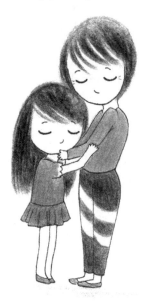

How does an eating disorder affect me?

The very behaviours of an eating disorder such as fasting, starvation, binge-eating and self-induced vomiting can result in serious physical complications such as dehydration, low blood sugar levels, electrolyte abnormalities, oesophageal rupture, hematemesis, gastritis and dental erosions. With prolonged malnutrition, stunting of growth, amenorrhea and subfertility, renal scarring, heart failure and cardiac arrhythmias, low bone density and in some severe cases neurocognitive deficits and cerebral atrophy and even death. As with most psychiatric conditions, the impact on psychosocial function can manifest in deteriorating academic performance, school refusal behaviours and social withdrawal. An older patient with the disorder may not be able to manage occupational demands, nor fulfil one's role as a spouse or parent.

I often notice that depression and anxiety symptoms co-exist with eating disorders and commonly manifest in patients feeling low and lacking in self-confidence, having negative self-thought, self-loathing and self-harm behaviours. Sometimes, anxiety symptoms manifest in the form of fear of eating in the company of others, anxiety in choosing foods or stepping up to certain food challenges. Some patients may also experience rigidity in the way food has to be prepared or served, or rigidity in the timing of meals. Some have developed an obsession to exercise or body checking.

How can I manage an eating disorder?

The first thing would be to tell someone about it. Opening up to a family member, a close friend, a teacher or a school counsellor could be the first step in the journey of managing the eating disorder. Verbalising it can help with assessing the extent of it, so as to determine the resources one may need to harness to get well. As stated above, eating disorders often come with a whole host of physiological and psychological implications, therefore it is recommended that one seeks professional help to manage the illness. A multi-pronged approach is often taken in management given the complex nature of the illness which impacts on various aspects of an individual, i.e., personal life and health, family life, romantic relationships, interpersonal relationships.

Nutritional management

In eating disorders, an integral part of treatment is to improve the nutritional status of the individual and regularise eating behaviours. Nutrition is crucial especially in patients with anorexia nervosa, with a focus towards a safe gradual increase in weight. For binge eating disorder and bulimia nervosa, while weight gain is not a core component of treatment, healthy nutrition remains important nonetheless as having consistent, regular, balanced eating habits help to reduce disordered eating behaviour. In anorexia nervosa, a prolonged restriction of food intake can lead to irreversible deterioration in various systems in the body, including the bones (osteoporosis), the brain and the reproductive system. Bone density and menses can be restored by weight gain alone. As such, meeting with a dietitian or a therapist who can help with nutritional intake is important, especially because some individuals may pose a risk for refeeding syndrome and need to be monitored professionally. A lot of the nutritional management is done in the home setting, so having a loved one who can be a part of the meal planning as well as provider of moral support for finishing meals is useful.

Psychological management

In patients with anorexia nervosa, the age of the individual is one of the factors that help determine what form of therapy may be most suitable. Family-based therapy centered on the Maudsley method has strong evidence in adolescents with anorexia nervosa, usually for a period of 6 months. This form of treatment requires the involvement of parents in managing the patient's meals during the process of refeeding. Separated family therapy where different members of the family are present at different points in time has also been shown to be better than combined family therapy when there are parents that display high forms of over-protectionism and criticism.

Other psychotherapeutic approaches to eating disorders include individual psychotherapy using elements from modalities such as (but not limited to) cognitive-behavioural therapy (CBT), psychodynamic therapy, interpersonal psychotherapy (IPT) and dialectical behaviour therapy (DBT). In such approaches, the patient meets with a psychotherapist on a regular basis to address the thoughts, behaviours and feelings associated with the eating disorder. The behaviours associated with eating disorders are a manifestation of deeper-seated issues which psychotherapy can help to uncover and work at. Contrary to popular belief, eating disorders are as little as possible to do with food and weight but a lot more to do with concepts of control, safety and predictability. Many individuals with eating disorders have developed them at a point in their life where they felt immensely out of control of events that happened to them and around them. For instance, if an individual is surrounded by relational instability at home where family members are constantly at loggerheads, he/she may feel like that aspect is not within his/her control, and may subconsciously turn toward controlling food intake and/or output as it is something that can be controlled. Likewise, someone who was sexually assaulted and felt out of control in that event may turn to controlling his/her food intake to regain a sense of safety. Speaking to a psychotherapist who is trained in understanding the mechanisms of an eating disorder can help in exploring, making sense of and processing the underlying causes. Eating disorders are also a means of communication — some individuals with eating disorders use their bodies and their behaviours to communicate what they are otherwise not able to communicate for various reasons. For instance, if there are broken channels of communication at home, a person may learn that he/she may only be able to communicate emotions (e.g., distress) or needs (attention/proximity-seeking) through the body. Some of our patients with anorexia nervosa have reflected to us that the only way they were able to cry for help was to *show* that they needed help, through maintaining a shockingly emaciated appearance. In this case, psychotherapy is also useful in helping one to identify his/her needs and also discovering healthy ways to communicate them.

In anorexia nervosa, individual psychotherapy is most useful when individuals are as close to their minimum healthy weight (weight-restored) as possible. This is due to the fact that cognitive rigidity hence the inability to take perspective persists when the individual is at a low weight, making the engagement in psychotherapy extremely difficult.

Art therapy

Art therapy is sometimes used in the management of eating disorders, particularly where there is potential for an individual to express through art the emotions that he/she otherwise cannot access, identify or verbalise.

What changes should I make to my daily activities now that I have an eating disorder?

Managing and recovering from an eating disorder can require certain lifestyle changes. For one, patients will need to set aside time to attend appointments with their healthcare professionals. This could mean rearranging their schedules to prioritise their health — some may have to miss classes or take time off work. Accepting that mental and physical wellness takes precedence over any other role or task is important.

Some individuals may have to put aside physical activity for a period of time — especially in the case of those with anorexia nervosa — to focus on weight gain and stabilising their vitals. In some cases, it may mean converting a run to a slow-paced walk, while in other cases it may mean remaining sedentary for a period of time. In the same thread, some students may have to be exempted from physical activity in school, as well as their extracurricular activities. While it may seem frustrating to have to sit out certain activities, it is only for a season! For those with bulimia nervosa or other eating disorders, a change in their exercise regime may also be required to manage an unhealthy obsession with exercise. Working toward a healthy and sustainable rhythm is the goal.

Prioritising mealtimes will be important, so as to regularise eating patterns. For some individuals, they may require practical support to get through mealtimes. This might mean that loved ones need to step in to accompany them during mealtimes for moral support, or that students are assigned teachers or school nurses to supervise their meals until they are ready to eat on their own again.

As individuals with eating disorders may be prone to comparing with others when it comes to weight, food, appearance or exercise, it may be useful for them to reduce potential unnecessary triggers. For example, it may be a good idea to identify certain social media accounts or platforms that can exacerbate unhelpful thoughts and remove access to them. Likewise, there may be unhelpful comments or activities in relation to one's social circle which may require some distancing from, especially during recovery. Developing an eating disorder as well as the process of relapsing can be a slippery slope — hence, it is not advisable for those living with an eating disorder or who have history of an eating disorder to go on diets/food fasts (even if it is for a reason other than weight loss), as one thing can easily lead to another. While dieting is a normalised phenomenon and most people who diet do not end up with an eating disorder, those who are prone to one may not be able to click the 'off' button and can end up spiralling into an unhealthy place. Therefore, eliminating certain foods entirely and labelling them as 'forbidden' is not the answer, rather, being able to eat anything and everything in moderation is key!

Recovering from an eating disorder is hard work, and can be an intense process with ups and downs. As such, individuals should ensure that they are engaging in self-care throughout the journey — treating themselves with utmost compassion and care on especially trying days and engaging in hobbies or activities they enjoy can lighten the load. As stress can exacerbate an eating disorder, reducing stress-inducing activities as well as learning to better cope with stress is important.

Ultimately, the aim is to shift the focus from food, weight and body image to other meaningful activities and goals in life. An eating disorder can take up a lot of head space and as such reduce a person's quality of life, oftentimes diminishing their sense of identity tied to anything other than the eating disorder. Recovering from an eating disorder, while daunting, can also be exciting and rewarding as one peels back the superficial layers of concerns and discovers things about oneself that propels him/her to a purposeful and enriching life.

SKIN DURING PUBERTY

Take Home Points

1. Puberty is a time of change and hormonal changes have a great influence on the condition of the skin and hair.
2. Morphological changes include the development of facial and body hair as secondary sex characteristics.
3. The skin gets oilier during puberty years and this can lead to acne which is the number one teenage skin problem experienced.
4. Pre-existing skin conditions such as eczema may get better or may be aggravated during these years.
5. Visible skin changes often cause significant concern for adolescents and may lead to significant emotional issues. Hence, understanding and anticipating these external changes is important.

Puberty is a time where the body goes through a myriad of changes and the skin is no exception. The skin is the largest organ in the body. From changes to the hair on your scalp, to the sweat glands in your feet, these head-to-toe changes can lead to a myriad of both physical and

---

Dr Angeline Yong is a Consultant Dermatologist and Dermatological Surgeon, specializing in skin cancer and Mohs micrographic surgery, hair disorders and hair transplantation, cosmetic dermatology and lasers, and is currently practising at Angeline Yong Dermatology, Gleneagles Medical Centre.

emotional issues; hence, understanding and anticipating these external changes is important for self-care and growing comfortable into one's skin.

Some of the obvious changes occur as a result of the hormonal changes that happen during the onset of puberty, as these changes result in the stimulation of certain glands in the skin, such as the sebaceous and eccrine glands. They also have a profound influence on how some common skin conditions such as eczema develop. Menstrual cycle hormonal fluctuations may actually give rise to a host of cutaneous changes including pre-menstrual exacerbation of these pre-existing skin conditions such as eczema and psoriasis.[1]

When does puberty start?

Puberty starts when a person's body matures from a child into that of an adult. It typically happens around ages 10 to 14 for girls, and 12 to 16 for boys. Do note that the time that puberty begins varies greatly among individuals, but usually occurs earlier in girls than boys. Other than genetics, environmental factors and body fat composition may play a role in the timing of puberty.

At this time, adolescents experience rapid growth and development of secondary sex characteristics, and certain skin conditions may worsen or first become apparent.[1]

Hair in new places. Why am I having increased body and facial hair growth?

Notable among the morphologic changes in the pubertal body is the development of secondary sex characteristics, and pertinent to the skin, is the development of pubic hair. In fact, puberty itself can be defined by 'pubarche' which is the appearance of pubic hair.

Before puberty, terminal hair is limited to the scalp, eyelashes and eyebrows. Following puberty, with the influence of androgens (mainly testosterone), terminal hair develops from vellus hair to give rise to secondary hair growth in the pubic regions and armpits).[2]

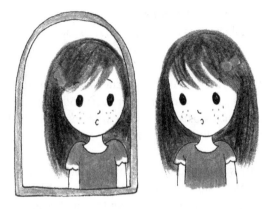

What are the common skin problems during puberty?

While puberty is a stage of life that everybody goes through, many medical conditions first appear during puberty. Some of the common skin conditions potentially associated with puberty are:

1. Acne
2. Hyperhidrosis
3. Axillary malodour (bromhidrosis)
4. Changes in congenital melanocytic nevi and congenital birthmarks
5. Eczema.[3]

Acne

Why are there zits on my face?

Acne is the most common skin problem occurring in teens. It ranges from small comedones (blackheads and whiteheads as we call them), to papules, pustules, nodules and cysts. Accompanying this may also be various forms of acne scarring such as red scars (post-inflammatory erythema), brown scars (post-inflammatory hyperpigmentation), and textural changes in the form of various types of depressed scars and even raised keloid scars.

Acne is an inflammation of the sebaceous glands which are found around the hair follicles of the skin. It is usually more pronounced over the face but may also occur over other sebaceous gland rich areas such as the scalp, back and chest. Hormonal changes at puberty lead to the activation of sebaceous glands and the subsequent development of acne in many adolescent boys and girls.

The main culprit when it comes to acne is testosterone. Testosterone is usually thought of as a male hormone, but everybody produces it to a certain extent. The amount of testosterone in our bodies increases during puberty, especially for boys. This is why acne is more common in teenage boys than in teenage girls.

This boost in testosterone levels during puberty can trigger acne as it makes the oil glands in our skin grow bigger. Some areas such as the scalp, face, back and upper chest are more prone to acne because they have pores that contain oil glands that produce the oily substance known as sebum. Sebum then gets secreted onto the surface of our skin to protect it. Overactivity of sebum production may block the pores with excess oil and dead skin cells, which in turn may attract bacteria that leads to redness and inflammation.[3,4]

When should I start cleansing my face and what sort of skincare routine should I look for?

Successful treatment of acne depends on the type of bumps an individual has and what skincare regimen has to be instituted to achieve the best results. In general:

- Acne-prone skin should be washed with a gentle cleanser and warm water one to two times per day. A cleanser containing a BHA like salicylic acid can be useful in the treatment of acne.
- Oil-free, non-comedogenic makeup, sun protection and moisturiser products should be used and makeup should be removed daily. Non-comedogenic refers to products that do not contain ingredients known to clog pores.
- Picking, squeezing or popping acne lesions (pimples) should be avoided.

Why do some teens get acne while others don't?

Acne is a very common problem during our teenage years. However, it does not affect everyone equally. Some teenagers have very clear skin with just occasional spots while others struggle with severe and widespread acne that requires treatment by a dermatologist.

80% of teenagers are affected by acne, with 3 in 10 teenagers having severe acne that has nodules and cysts that will lead to scarring. Whilst teenage acne can last for 5 to 10 years without treatment and usually disappears by the early 20s, some teenage acne can go on into adulthood.

Why some teenagers have more acne compared to others may be due to a myriad of factors including genetics (severe acne seems to run in some families), differences in testosterone levels, usage of greasy products or too much cosmetics on the skin, and taking certain kinds of medications.

Does diet play a role?

Acne has been linked closely to high fat and sugary foods. A teenage diet that is stereotypically rich in sugary drinks and junk food can create a surge in cell signalling, which stimulates grease production in the skin, as well as inflammation, ultimately leading to acne. Dairy products is another postulated factor. Avoiding overconsumption of ice-creams, cheese and other dairy-based food is important. A healthy, balanced diet is essential for keeping skin healthy and glowing.

What are possible treatments I can try on my own?

There are many over-the-counter products for prevention and treatment of acne. Products with benzoyl peroxide and salicylic acid are highly effective in treating most mild forms of acne. Benzoyl peroxide kills skin bacteria that can lead to acne and also reduces inflammation associated with pimples. Salicylic acid treats acne by causing the skin to dry out and peel, and reduces swelling.

It is also important to note that acne medications typically take weeks or months to work, so do not expect to see instant or same-day results. Avoid impatience and subsequent polypharmacy which can lead to further skin irritation and the development of concurrent facial dermatitis, as products used for the treatment of acne can often cause dryness and irritation when used excessively and when layered one after another.

If your acne does not get better with over-the-counter products, seeking medical help would be useful. If you are still struggling to manage your acne, make sure you consult a dermatologist who can develop a bespoke treatment plan for you. Doctors can prescribe other topicals such as retinoid creams, azelaic acid and antibiotics such as clindamycin and erythromycin creams which can be helpful in the management of the acne. In addition, oral medications ranging from antibiotics like doxycycline, isotretinoin, and hormonal medications for those with concurrent irregular periods may be beneficial for suitable individuals. External treatment options with blue light LED, chemical peels, extractions and medical grade facials, and certain lasers may also be useful.

Hyperhidrosis

Help! Why am I sweaty all the time?

Be it on the palms of your hands or soles of your feet, underarms, or anywhere on your body, you are not alone if you often find yourself drenched in perspiration. Excess sweating is a major issue for many teens. The increase in various hormones during puberty may also make the sweat glands more active.[3,4]

What are some tips to reduce symptoms?

Consider wearing clothing with natural fibres like cotton, which are cooler and more absorbent. Wear socks and try to alternate shoes so that they can dry out. Avoid foods and drinks that seem to trigger sweating such as spicy dishes, or very hot liquids such as soups.

Can this be treated?

A topical antiperspirant can help to reduce perspiration output, and these agents work by plugging the sweat ducts so the perspiration does not reach the skin.

However, when heavy sweating occurs on a regular basis, you may be experiencing what doctors call 'hyperhidrosis'. This condition is characterised by excessive sweating on the palms, soles, underarms, and sometimes even the face. If topical antiperspirant does not help, seek medical help and advice as a range of other options ranging from iontophoresis, botox injections and oral medications can be used to alleviate some of these symptoms. This is especially if you are experiencing functional problems especially with the grip on the hands and the symptoms are exerting real impact on your daily activities such as writing, playing a musical instrument, or sports.

Bromhirosis

Is it me or do I smell different?

While sweat is actually odourless, the body odour associated with sweat results from bacteria on the skin multiplying in sweaty areas like armpits and breaking down the sweat into amino acids.

Showering or bathing with soap removes the bacteria that causes body odour, so a daily shower or bath with soap and water — paying particular attention to the armpit area, genital area and feet — is key. Deodorant helps keep the body smelling fresh once the bacteria has been removed. Topical antiperspirants can help decrease sweating, so using a deodorant/antiperspirant combo is also helpful. Apply each morning and keep on hand to re-apply during times of increased physical activity.[3,4]

Changing Moles and Birthmarks

Is my mole changing and getting darker?

Congenital melanocytic nevus (brown birthmarks) tend to increase in size and become more pigmented during puberty. Prominent terminal hairs may also start to form and grow within then. Sebaceous naevi also typically become thicker with a more raised, bumpy surface.

If there are significant changes in the size and colour of the moles, seek advice from your medical practitioner on whether this may be cause for concern and if close monitoring or a biopsy may be needed.

Eczema

Does eczema get better or worse?

This is a common question posed by many parents when we see young children with eczema or atopic dermatitis. Although more commonly seen in younger children, some children actually 'outgrow' eczema with the hormonal changes that start during puberty. However, some kids continue to experience these patches of dry, scaly, reddened skin into their teen years and the severity may even be aggravated during this time. Teens who are active in sports may actually find that their childhood eczema worsens, frequently aggravated by trauma or by sporting equipment which can lead to frictional aggravation.

Sometimes a fragrance-free moisturiser is all you need. This is especially important if you are frequently in dry air-conditioned environments, or swim frequently. Applying the moisturising lotion within 10 minutes after bathing helps to lock in the moisture best.

If a moisturiser does not help and the skin remains weepy or oozy, and is significantly red or itchy, it may be time to see a family practitioner or dermatologist who can prescribe medications such as appropriate strength steroid creams, antibiotics or even non-steroidal class anti-inflammatory creams which will help. Occasionally, oral medications or even newer-class injection form medications known as 'biologics' may be used by the dermatologist if the condition is severe enough to warrant it.

In summary, the teenage years are a sensitive time for all, as we try to 'grow into our own skin'. Self-esteem and confidence issues are certainly part and parcel of life as we grapple with developing our own identity. During this rapid physical development, the perception of others may hold significant influence on the way we view ourselves, hence understanding and anticipating these external changes is important for the mental health and well-being of every young teen.[3,4]

References

1.   Biro FM and Chan Y-M. Normal Puberty. UpToDate; 2014. Available at: https://www.uptodate.com/contents/normal-puberty.
2.   Messenger AD, de Berker BA, and Sinclair RD. Disorders of hair. In *Rook's Textbook of Dermatology* (8th Edition), eds. Burns T, Breathnach S, Cox N, Griffiths C. Oxford, UK: Blackwell (2010).
3.   Millington GWM, and Graham-Browne RAC. Skin and skin disease throughout life. In *Rook's Textbook of Dermatology* (8th Edition), eds. Burns T, Breathnach S, Cox N, Griffiths C. Oxford, UK: Blackwell (2010).
4.   Wong D. Skin Changes at Puberty. Dermnetnz; 2014 Dec. Available at: https://dermnetnz.org/topics/skin-changes-at-puberty.

YOUNG WOMANHOOD

CONTRACEPTION AND FAMILY PLANNING

Take Home Points

1. There is no 100 percent safe and effective family planning method. The choice of method depends on your preferences and the pros and cons of the method that is most ideal for your situation, which may change over time.
2. A discussion with your partner and doctor is important in choosing the right method for you. The doctor will assess your health risks and possible interactions between the contraception and your medical conditions or medications you are taking.
3. Methods for short-term and long-term family planning are available. In general, short-term methods rely on you taking medication regularly, while long-term methods consist of devices that can be inserted into the womb or arm to release medication slowly over the years.
4. Using two methods of birth control together should offer better protection than one method alone, so using condoms is highly encouraged together with whichever other method you have

---

(Continued)

Dr Janice Tung is a Consultant Obstetrician and Gynaecologist, specializing in Reproductive Medicine, and is currently practising at the O&G Specialist Clinic, Thomson Fertility Centre.

(Continued)

> chosen. Condoms also have the added benefit of reducing the risk of sexually transmitted infections.
> 5. You should be familiar with the risks and benefits of the method you have chosen and know what to expect, how to monitor for risks and what to do in the event of unwanted side effects.

What is contraception?

Most women can become pregnant from the time they reach puberty in their teens until they begin menopause in their late 40s or early 50s. Birth control, or contraception, allows a woman and her partner to minimise the risk of an unwanted pregnancy, and plan the number and spacing of children they want. A woman may get pregnant at any time in her period cycle although there are some days where chance of pregnancy may be lower or higher (NO DAY IS SAFE!). A woman without regular periods or with previous apparent difficulty in getting pregnant may also get pregnant anytime naturally, and should also consider contraception if they do not want pregnancy.

What are the various contraceptive options?

Birth control can be achieved by permanent and non-permanent methods.

Permanent methods

As the name suggests, these are not reversible, and are suitable for couples who are certain that they do not want children anymore. A common misconception is that permanent equals 100% effectiveness, but that is not true. They involve clipping or sealing off both the fallopian tubes in the woman, or sealing off both sperm ducts in the man. There is still a small chance of failure of the method to prevent pregnancy (<1 percent).

Non-permanent methods

These may be suitable for young women who want to be sexually active but delay their first pregnancies or space out their children. The option remains open for future pregnancies, i.e., they may stop using the method when they wish to get pregnant. Non-permanent methods can be hormonal or non-hormonal, short-term or long-term.

No birth control or contraceptive method is absolutely 100 percent effective. Only abstinence from sex ensures no risk of pregnancy.

Which method is right for me?

Each birth control method has good points as well as potential side-effects. A couple may find one method suits them better than others, depending on their needs and preferences. These may change over time. Using two methods of birth control together (for example, condoms and oral contraceptive pill) may offer better protection than one method alone. A method may also not be suitable for certain women depending on their personal and family history of medical conditions. For example, women with a tendency towards migraine attacks would not be suitable for oral contraceptives. Some methods may also have additional benefits aside from birth control, e.g., oral contraceptives can also help to reduce heavy menstrual flow.

Bear in mind, there is no 100 percent ideal method. Each option comes with its risks and benefits, and couples should have a discussion with their doctors in order to decide which option is most suitable for and acceptable to them.

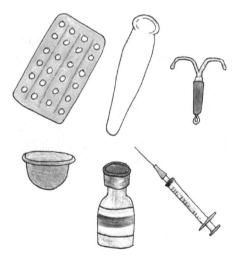

What are the commonly used methods of contraception?

Barrier methods

1. Condom

This is one of the most common methods for contraception and is readily available at retail stores. It is a disposable thin, latex sheath, which is rolled directly over the erect penis before sex, and it should be removed after withdrawing the penis from the vagina, before the penis becomes soft. When used correctly and consistently, and together with spermicide creams, it is about 90 percent reliable in preventing pregnancy. Condoms also have the added benefit of reducing the risk of sexually transmitted infections. However, some people may be sensitive to latex.

2. Diaphragm

This is a soft, shallow latex dome that is placed over the cervix inside the vagina before sex. This helps to prevent sperm from entering through the cervix, and it is usually used together with spermicide creams. A good fit is required. Some ladies may find it difficult to position the diaphragm correctly.

Short-term hormonal methods

3. Combined oral contraceptive pill (the pill)

The pill contains a mixture of female hormones called oestrogen and progestogen and should be taken every day, at approximately the same time. It works by preventing the release of the female egg, thickening the cervical mucus and changing the surface of the womb lining to make it unsuitable for pregnancy. When taken correctly and regularly, this method is 98 to 99 percent reliable. Some medications and herbs such as antibiotics and St John's wort may interact with the pill and reduce its effectiveness. There are different regimens: 21 days of taking the hormone pill and 7 days of being 'hormone-free', as well as 24 'pill' days with 4 'pill-free' days. Once stopped, it may take a couple of cycles before you can become pregnant.

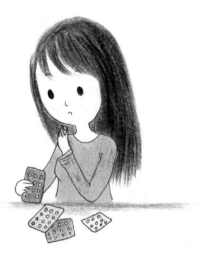

Who is it suitable for?

Oral contraceptives are popular among young women who are looking for shorter term birth control and not likely to forget pills, or who may also wish to regulate their menstruation. This method is not suitable for ladies who are fully breastfeeding for the first 6 months post-delivery.

There are also other benefits to taking oral contraceptives, although they would not be taken expressly for these reasons. Pill users have a lower risk of ovarian and womb cancers.

What side effects are there?

Short-term side effects include skin changes such as acne, mood changes, breast tenderness and nausea, which may improve after 2–3 months. Some ladies may experience decreased libido. Long-term side effects are uncommon and occur in older women who are taking them. These include the risk of aggravating cardiovascular conditions, such as heart attack or stroke. Hence, this method is not suitable for women with a history of these conditions.

There is no increased risk of breast cancer. As the pill is usually avoided in ladies above 45 years old, a lady in her 50s who had been on the pill in the past will not be at any increased risk of breast cancer compared with another lady in her 50s who had never been on the pill. This method would not be suitable for those with a history of liver problems, migraine attacks, or epilepsy who are on certain types of anti-epileptic medications.

Very rarely, there is a risk of thromboembolism, which is a potentially life-threatening condition where blood clots form in big veins in the legs, which may travel up to the veins in the lungs, causing chest pain, breathlessness and collapse. This risk is highest in the first year of pill usage, and falls thereafter. However, the risk is unpredictable in the sense that many will not have a family or personal history of this condition. If you do, this method is not suitable for you. If you develop this while taking the pill, it will be more likely to happen if you fall pregnant. Such ladies will require special precautions during pregnancy for prevention of blood clots.

4.   Progestogen-only contraceptive pill (mini pill)

This contains only one type of female hormone — progestogen, as its name implies. It is less reliable than the pill. It has to be taken every day strictly and can be taken by breastfeeding mothers. It works by thickening cervical mucus and preventing the release of female eggs from the ovaries but is less effective than the combined oral contraceptive pill. It has no or minimal risks of stroke and blood clotting in comparison to the combined oral contraceptive pill. Once stopped, it may take a couple of cycles before you can become pregnant.

5.   Hormonal patch

The hormonal patch comes as a small adhesive patch that is worn on certain parts of the body every day and night. It is changed every week for three weeks, followed by a break of one week with no patch. It releases the same female hormones oestrogen and progestogen as the combined oral contraceptive pill through the skin into the bloodstream, to prevent the release of the female egg, thicken the cervical mucus and change the surface of the womb lining to make it unsuitable for pregnancy. It is suitable for ladies who would like to use the combined oral contraceptive pill, but have concerns about remembering to take a pill at the same time every day and do not mind having a patch on the skin. Some ladies may develop an irritation or allergic skin reaction to the patch. The same uses, side effects and contraindications as the combined oral contraceptive pill applies.

6. Progestogen-only injection

The hormone, progestogen, is injected directly into the muscle where it slowly enters the bloodstream over a period of time. It works by thickening the cervical mucus and preventing the release of female eggs from the ovaries. It provides contraception for 12 to 14 weeks at a time, and is more than 99 percent reliable. It is suitable for ladies who want a cheap, effective way of preventing pregnancy for an intermediate period of time. It may result in irregular bleeding patterns, although more than 80 percent of ladies will have no periods after the first 3 to 4 injections. It may result in weight gain. Taking it for more than 2 years may give rise to accelerated bone loss which is reversible after stopping the medication, so taking it long-term is not suitable for ladies at risk of osteoporosis. Once stopped, it can take up to a year for periods and chance of pregnancy to return.

Long-term hormonal methods

7. Hormonal intrauterine device (e.g., Mirena)

This is a device that is inserted into the womb by a doctor in the clinic so as to provide long-term contraception for up to 5 years. The hormone progestogen is released directly in the womb slowly over 5 years. This causes the lining to be unsuitable for pregnancy and partially prevents ovulation. It is more than 99 percent reliable. Although rare, if the device fails and the lady gets pregnant with it still inside the womb, there is a risk of the pregnancy being located outside the womb (ectopic pregnancy) which is potentially dangerous and may require medical or surgical treatment.

The main unwanted side effect from the device is irregular or erratic bleeding patterns, which if heavy and bothersome, may cause ladies to have the device removed prematurely before 5 years. The device has a thread that may be seen at the cervix to help remove it. However sometimes, this cannot be seen in the clinic at the time of removal, and the retained device may have to be removed via a small surgical procedure with a scope instead. In some cases, the device may drop out prematurely without notice, and the lady may become pregnant if she is unaware that she is no longer on contraception. There is also a small risk of womb infection within the first 6 weeks of inserting the device.

8. Hormonal implants in the arm (e.g., Implanon)

This device is inserted on the inner aspect of your upper arm slightly above the elbow, and may be changed every 3 years in a procedure performed in the clinic. It may be felt deliberately under the skin, but otherwise, is usually unnoticeable. It releases the hormone progestogen slowly over 3 years. It works by thickening cervical mucus and preventing the release of female eggs from the ovaries. It is almost 100 percent reliable since there is no risk of it dropping out.

The main unwanted side effect from the device is irregular or erratic bleeding patterns, which if heavy and bothersome, may cause ladies to have the device removed prematurely before 3 years. It may also result in weight gain.

Long-term non-hormonal method

9.   Copper Intrauterine Device (IUCD)

This is a device that is inserted in the womb by a doctor in the clinic so as to provide long-term contraception from 3 to 5 years. It works by causing a chemical change that damages the sperm and the egg before they can meet and making the womb lining unsuitable for implantation. It is 98 to 99 percent reliable. Although rare, if the device fails and the lady gets pregnant with it still inside the womb, there is a risk of the pregnancy being located outside the womb (ectopic pregnancy) which is potentially dangerous and may require medical or surgical treatment.

The method is non-hormonal, and as such, your bleeding pattern will not be affected by this method. However, a lady may experience heavier and more painful periods with this device, especially if she already had heavy and painful periods to begin with. The device has a thread that may be seen at the cervix to help remove it. However sometimes, this cannot be seen in the clinic at the time of removal, and the retained device may have to be removed via a small surgical procedure with a scope instead. In some ladies, the device may drop out prematurely without notice, and the lady may become pregnant if she is unaware that she is no longer on contraception. There is also a small risk of womb infection within the first 6 weeks of inserting the device.

CERVICAL CANCER AND SCREENING

Take Home Points

1. Cervical cancer is the second most common cancer in women worldwide and is mostly caused by the HPV virus.
2. Cervical cancer is easily prevented by regular PAP smears and/or HPV testing.
3. Every sexually active woman should undergo a PAP smear screen at least once in every 3 years.
4. HPV vaccination is an effective way to prevent cervical cancer. However, HPV vaccinations do not replace the need for regular PAP smears.
5. An abnormal PAP smear can be easily treated if diagnosed early.

Dr Freda Khoo is a Consultant Obstetrician and Gynaecologist, in General Obstetrics and Gynaecology, and is currently practising at Thomson Medical Centre.

Why do I need to do a PAP smear?

A PAP smear is done to pick up early cervical abnormal or pre-cancerous cells, so that we can more closely monitor the condition. If need be, we can thoroughly treat the disease before it progresses into full-fledged cancer. If the cervical pre-cancer is picked up early, it can be fully treatable.

What happens during a PAP smear?

During a PAP smear, you will be asked to lie down on the doctor's examination couch. Your doctor will pass a plastic speculum into your vagina to open up the walls of your vagina so that your doctor can see your cervix.

Upon visualisation of your cervix, a small broom-like brush will then be used to pick up cells from the surface of your cervix. These cells will be mixed into a solution and sent to the laboratory for testing.

What results can I expect from a PAP smear?

The PAP smear results typically take around one week to be out. The results can be normal, or reported as Cervical Intraepithelial Neoplasia (CIN), which is the scientific term for cervical pre-cancer. Some other terms which may be found in a PAP smear report include ASCUS (Atypical Squamous Cell of Unknown Significance) and ASC-H (Atypical Squamous cells — wherein High-grade Squamous Intraepithelial lesion cannot be ruled out). Your doctor or gynaecologist will explain the significance of the results to you.

At times, signs of infection with the Human Papilloma Virus (HPV) may be seen in the cells, and thus reflected in the report.

What is the cause of abnormal PAP smear results?

The Human Papilloma Virus (HPV) is the culprit for causing abnormal PAP smears. We get infected with HPV through sexual contact. It could be from sexual intercourse or heavy petting. Because the HPV is a virus, there is no medication to take to treat the HPV infection.

We have to rely on our immune system to clear the HPV infection. If the HPV infection fails to be cleared, the HPV will work on the cells of the surface of the cervix, and cause them to change. Over a period of a few years, normal cells will turn into pre-cancer cells, and if untreated, the pre-cancer cells may eventually turn into cancer cells after 5 to 10 more years.

There are many different HPV subtypes — as many as more than 150. The different HPV subtypes are grouped into 3 groups — low, potentially high, and high-risk types.

It is the high-risk subtypes of HPV, particularly HPV 16 and 18, that cause cervical pre-cancer and cancer changes.

Are there any other risks for getting cervical cancer or pre-cancer?

There are some risk factors which may increase the risk of getting cervical cancer or pre-cancer, namely:

— Smoking
— First intercourse at a young age
— Having or having had multiple sexual partners
— Having a partner who has other sexual partners
— History of sexually transmitted diseases
— HIV infection
— Oral contraceptive use of greater than 5 years
— Nutritional deficiency
— Birthing 3 or more children
— Genetic factors.

When then, do I need to do a PAP smear?

Under the Singapore National Cervical Cancer Screening Programme that has been implemented through the polyclinics, if you have ever been sexually active and are between 25 and 29 years old, you should have a PAP smear at least every 3 years. If you are between 30 and 69 years old, you should have a HPV test at least every 5 years. After 69 years of age, you do not need to attend screening anymore.

Other options for screening (not under the Singapore National Cervical Cancer Screening Programme) include:

— Doing a PAP smear at least every 3 years
— Doing a HPV test at least every 5 years
— Doing a PAP smear and HPV test at least every 5 years.

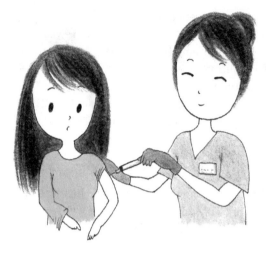

I have received cervical cancer vaccination. Do I still need to undergo PAP smears?

Cervical cancer vaccinations only work to prevent future infections of HPV. That means that if you have been infected with the HPV virus before vaccination, the vaccination would not be able to cure or eradicate the virus. Also, vaccinations do not have a 100 percent guarantee of preventing HPV infections.

Thus, even if you have been vaccinated, you should still undergo regular PAP smears or HPV testing. The HPV vaccine is not a substitute for cervical cancer screening.

Should I still get a HPV vaccination then?

HPV vaccination is an effective way of preventing HPV infection, and thus cervical cancers. Thus, it is recommended for ladies to receive the HPV vaccination. It is best taken when one is sexually naïve — before one's first sexual experience. However, if one is already currently sexually active and has not been vaccinated, the vaccine is still certainly helpful in preventing future disease.

Although the vaccine is licensed for girls and women from 9 to 26 years old, there is also evidence that the benefit of the vaccine can be extended to women older than 26 years old.

There are currently 3 vaccines available in Singapore. Cervarix protects against 2 subtypes of HPV, Gardasil protects against 4 subtypes of HPV, and Gardasil-9 protects against 9 subtypes of HPV.

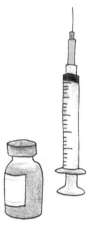

I have an abnormal PAP smear. What does that mean?

Most importantly, DO NOT PANIC! This is exactly the reason for PAP smears — to be able to pick up abnormal pre-cancerous results before they silently turn into full-fledged cancer.

An abnormal PAP smear just means that the cells on the surface of your cervix have started to turn abnormal due to them being infected with the Human Papilloma Virus (HPV). If the problem persists, it may progress to cervical cancer in the long term, 10 to 20 years down the road.

What is the next step when I receive the result of an abnormal PAP smear?

When you get an abnormal PAP smear, you will be referred to a gynaecologist. You might be required to take further tests for HPV infection. Or, you might require a more in-depth examination. This is called a colposcopy examination.

During a colposcopy examination, you will lie on a couch, and the doctor will look at your cervix in greater detail under a microscope, to further confirm the findings of the abnormal PAP smear.

If any abnormality is found in the Colposcopic examination, your doctor may take some biopsies from your cervix to be sent to the laboratory for confirmation.

I have been diagnosed with cervical cancer. What is next?

If you have been diagnosed with cervical cancer, you will have to be referred to a gynae-oncologist. You will then be required to undergo a series of scans to ascertain the extent of spread of the cancer. You will also need to undergo an examination under anaesthesia, to examine if the surrounding organs have been invaded by the cancer.

Your gynae-oncologist will then most likely plan for a surgery for you. Thereafter, the need to undergo radiotherapy and chemotherapy depends on a few factors, among them would be the stage of the disease, the subtype of the cancer and the extent of local invasion.

Further Reading

Basic Information about Cervical Cancer. Centers for Disease Control and Prevention; 2021 Jan. Available at: https://www.cdc.gov/cancer/cervical/basic_info/.

Cervical Screening: Programme and Colposcopy Management. The British Society for Colposcopy and Cervical Pathology; 2020. Available at: https://www.bsccp.org.uk/healthcare-professionals/professional-news/publication-of-updated-cervical-screening-programme-and-colposcopy-manageme/.

Management Guidelines for Cervical Screening and Preinvasive Disease of the Cervix. Cervical Screen Singapore Advisory Committee; 2019 Feb. Available at: https://www.sccps.org/wp-content/uploads/2019/03/CSS-Clinical-Mgt-Guidelines-2019_March-Release.pdf.

Scientific Committee Position Paper on HPV Vaccination. The Society for Colposcopy and Cervical Pathology of Singapore; 2020 Mar. Available at: https://www.sccps.org/wp-content/uploads/2020/03/SCCPS-Scientific-Committee-Position-Paper-on-HPV-Vaccination-Final.pdf.

Scientific Committee Position Paper on Primary HPV Screening for Cervical Cancer Prevention. The Society for Colposcopy and Cervical Pathology of Singapore; 2016 Mar. Available at: https://www.sccps.org/wp-content/uploads/2018/03/SCCPS-Scientific-Committee-Position-Paper-on-HPV-Screening.pdf.

STARTING A FAMILY

EFFECTS OF PREGNANCY ON THE BODY

Take Home Points

1. Many profound changes occur to all the organs in your body as you embark on your pregnancy journey.
2. Nausea, breast tenderness, skin changes, constipation, backache and fatigue are just a few of the many physical changes you may experience during pregnancy.
3. Although your body increases its energy requirements during pregnancy, "eating for two" is not advisable as it may cause excessive weight gain in pregnancy.
4. Keeping active during pregnancy can have many benefits, but certain exercises such as hot yoga or contact sports should best be avoided.
5. Certain symptoms such as severe itchiness, shortness of breath and unilateral leg swelling may be the result of an underlying medical condition. If you feel unwell, you should highlight your symptoms to your doctor.

Dr Celene Hui is a Consultant Obstetrician and Gynaecologist in the Minimally Invasive Surgery Unit, and is currently practising at the KK Women's and Children's hospital. She is also a Clinical Assistant Professor at Duke-NUS Medical School.

Pregnancy is an amazing journey that brings about many profound changes to all the organs in your body. Many of these changes occur soon after fertilisation and continue throughout the pregnancy, as a response to the stimuli from your baby and the placenta.

How does my womb change during pregnancy?

In a non-pregnant woman, the womb or uterus is approximately the size of an orange, weighing about 70g. During pregnancy, the muscle cells of the uterus grow and multiply in response to the hormones of pregnancy and the mechanical stretching from your growing baby. Around 12 weeks of pregnancy, your uterus would become the size of a grapefruit and at around 20 weeks, it would reach the level of your belly button. Your doctor would be able to measure the distance between your pubic bone and the top of your uterus known as the fundus. By the end of your pregnancy, the uterus would have transformed into a much larger organ weighing almost 1100g. After birth, your uterus will slowly shrink over 6 weeks to return to its pre-pregnancy size and this process is called involution.

How does my cervix change during pregnancy?

The cervix is a firm, cylindrical structure at the lower part of the uterus and it plays an integral role in maintaining and protecting your pregnancy. A special thick mucus produced by the cervix acts as a 'plug' at the entrance of the uterus, rich in substances that act as an immunological barrier to protect your baby against ascending infection from the vagina. Part of the lining of the cervix contains glands that produce this mucus. Cervical ectropion in pregnancy is when these glands grow larger and extend outwards onto the surface, resulting in the surface of the cervix becoming redder and more prone to bleeding. Despite the mechanical forces acting upon it by your growing baby, the cervix must remain closed throughout the pregnancy. Weakening or shortening of the cervix can lead to pregnancy loss in the second trimester or preterm birth.

How will my breasts change during pregnancy?

From early on in your pregnancy, you may notice your breasts becoming more sensitive and tender. This is in response to the rising hormones in pregnancy as well as the increased blood flow to your breasts. Your breasts will also continue to grow in size during the pregnancy and it is normal to go up a bra cup size or two. Interestingly, a larger pre-pregnancy breast size does not equate to a subsequent higher volume of milk production.

The areolae are the circles of pigmented skin around your nipples. Both your nipples and areolae will enlarge and darken during your pregnancy. The appearance of bumps on the areolae, or Montgomery's tubercles, become more pronounced. You may also notice nipple discharge when the breasts are stimulated during pregnancy. Breast lumps in pregnancy are common and may be due to clogged milk ducts, lipomas, fibroadenomas, cysts or accessory breast tissue. However, it is advisable to highlight a newly discovered breast lump to your doctor as it can be the first presentation of breast cancer, though such cases are rare.

After delivery, the nipples express a thick yellowish fluid called colostrum. Compared with mature milk, colostrum contains more minerals, amnio acids and protein but less sugar and fat. It also contains antibodies, and its content of immunoglobulin A (IgA) offers your new born baby protection against certain gut bacterial infections. Over the next few days after delivery, your breasts will produce milk instead of colostrum. Breast milk is a special mélange of nutrients, antibodies and bacteria, rich in benefits for your baby. Emerging studies suggest that bacteria from breast milk and breastfeeding can help to shape the gut microbiome of your baby in early life, and this may have an impact on his or her long-term health.

What are the skin changes to expect in pregnancy?

Expectant mothers often radiate a luminous 'pregnancy glow'. Greater blood volume and improved blood circulation result in the skin looking pink and flushed. Changes in the hormone levels also cause the sebaceous glands of the face to secrete more oil or sebum, resulting in a shiny and supple skin appearance. The downside is that excess sebum may make you more prone to acne during your pregnancy.

Nine out of ten women will experience darkening of their skin during pregnancy. You may notice a dark, brownish-black line called the *linea nigra* appearing in the midline of your abdomen, from your belly button to your pubic area. Occasionally, you may experience dark patches appearing on your face, giving rise to what is known as the 'mask of pregnancy'. These uneven patches are worsened by exposure to sunlight, so a good broad-spectrum UVA/UVB sunscreen should be used daily. Darkening of moles, freckles and birthmarks can also occur during pregnancy and these hyperpigmentation changes usually fade or lighten considerably after delivery. Although common, it is always advisable to inform your doctor if you notice any changes in the colour, shape or size of any skin lesions.

Stretch marks are extremely common and are caused by the breakage of the elastic fibres just under the surface of the skin. Stretch marks often begin as pink or violet patches in the sixth and seventh months of pregnancy and evolve into indented streaks or lines that are lighter in colour. These marks are more common on the tummy, thighs and breasts. Some women are more prone to getting stretch marks than others, and studies have shown the strongest associated risk factors to be excessive maternal weight gain, young maternal age and family history. Unfortunately, there is no way to prevent the development of stretch marks completely. Many lotions and creams can be used to improve the hydration and elasticity of the skin to better withstand the stretching process, while avoiding excessive sudden weight gain in your pregnancy may be helpful.

Is it normal to experience itching in pregnancy?

Mild itching in pregnancy can be due to the increased blood supply to the skin as well as the skin stretching over the abdomen. Pregnancy increases your basal body temperature and causes you to perspire more, making you more prone to heat rash and hives. Heat rash can cause an itchy, prickly patch on your skin while hives can cause itchy raised bumps. Stretch marks, as mentioned earlier, can also feel itchy. A particular itchy rash specific to pregnancy called PUPPP, pruritic urticarial papules and plagues of pregnancy, can develop as the skin stretches. Your doctor can recommend creams to soothe dry, itchy or inflamed skin.

It is worthy to note that a condition called obstetric cholestasis which affects the liver also presents the symptom of itching. The itching of obstetric cholestasis usually begins in the third trimester, starting from the palms of your hands and soles of your feet and spreading to the rest of your body. It often disturbs sleep as it is worse at night. Sometimes, itching is the only clue that may make your doctor suspect you have obstetric cholestasis. It is important to detect this condition as it has implications on the well-being of your baby. Obstetric cholestasis increases the risk of your baby being born premature or your pregnancy resulting in a stillbirth.

Why is my hair thicker during my pregnancy?

During pregnancy, you may find that your scalp hair is at its thickest and shiniest. This is because the hormone oestrogen slows the normal progression from the anagen hair growth phase to the telogen resting phase. Sometimes, you may even find that you have excessive hair growth in other unwanted areas like your face or belly. These effects are not permanent. Approximately one to four months after birth, you may suddenly experience an abrupt loss of hair, with an alarming amount of hair being shed just with combing or washing. Rest assured that this is only temporary and your normal hair growth would resume in 6 to 12 months.

How does pregnancy affect my heart?

Many changes occur to your circulatory system from the moment your pregnancy begins to adapt to the increased demand of oxygen and nutrients from your growing baby and womb. These changes can put stress on a woman's heart during pregnancy and may sometimes unmask underlying heart conditions.

During pregnancy, there is a decrease in the resistance of blood flowing through your blood vessels, resulting in a drop in blood pressure. Your heart rate will rise from the first trimester, averaging between 10 to 30 beats higher than your pre-pregnancy heart rate. Overall, the cardiac output, or the amount of blood being pumped by the heart, increases by 30 to 50 percent. This value increases even further during labour. Your heart works harder during pregnancy and you may experience some irregularities in heart rhythm. As your uterus size increases past the level of the belly button, it can also compress on the large blood vessel leading from the lower body to the heart known as the inferior vena cava. This compression decreases blood flow to and from the heart, and can cause sudden dizziness or fainting spells when you stand up from a lying down or sitting down position.

During pregnancy the plasma in your blood increases by 40 to 50 percent while the number of red blood cells increases by 20 to 30 percent. This disproportionate increase results in a physiological drop in your haemoglobin level during pregnancy, or dilutional anaemia. This anaemia is further exacerbated by the transfer of iron stores from you to your baby. Hence, you are advised to increase your iron intake during pregnancy.

Is it normal to feel breathless during my pregnancy?

Many changes occur within the respiratory system during pregnancy. There is a greater oxygen demand due to a higher metabolic rate and a 20 percent increase in the consumption of oxygen. The pregnancy hormone progesterone stimulates your brain to increase the frequency and depth of your breaths, so you take in more oxygen by hyperventilating. During pregnancy, the circumference of your rib cage also increases and the enlarging uterus causes an upward displacement of the diaphragm. Together with the awareness of hyperventilation, these can lead to a pregnant woman having an increased sensation of breathlessness or 'air hunger'. Breathlessness during pregnancy occurs in up to three in four pregnant women at some point in their pregnancies. You may feel breathless at rest or while talking and there may be paradoxical improvement with mild activity.

Although feeling breathless is common and is a normal physiological change in pregnancy, it may also be the consequence of other life-threatening medical conditions. A blood clot in the lung (known as pulmonary embolism), lung infection or even excessive fluid in the lungs due to heart failure can also present with breathlessness in pregnancy and will require immediate medical attention. If your shortness of breath is severe, causing difficulty in lying flat, or associated with other symptoms such as fever or painful swelling of the legs, you should consult your doctor.

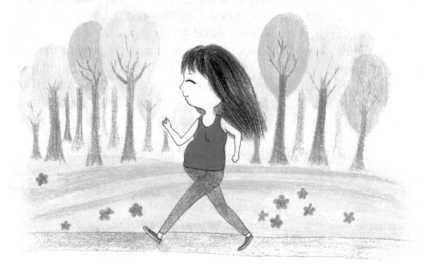

Can I exercise during pregnancy?

There are many benefits to staying active during pregnancy, including reducing back pain, easing constipation, reducing your risk of getting gestational diabetes and improving your overall fitness and strength. However, the increased stress on the heart and lungs during pregnancy can affect your ability to exercise. The increasing size of your uterus, lax ligaments, and changes in posture and sense of balance can further contribute to difficulties in exercising. Brisk walking and swimming are safe exercises recommended in pregnancy. If you have certain medical disorders or pregnancy complications, your doctor may advise you against exercising. Any sport that may result in a rise in body temperature such as hot yoga or any trauma to the abdomen such as contact sports, should best be avoided.

Why do I feel nauseous during my pregnancy?

Although 'morning sickness' is the common term used for mild pregnancy related nausea and vomiting, you may experience symptoms at any time of the day. Nausea and vomiting in pregnancy often begins from the fifth to sixth weeks of pregnancy, peaking at 10 to 12 weeks and typically improving by 16 weeks. It affects 5 to 9 in 10 pregnant women and the severity of symptoms can vary. This can be attributed to the increase in pregnancy hormones and the slowing down of the movement of gastric contents. A small percentage of pregnant women may continue to feel nauseous for the rest of their pregnancy until delivery.

Avoiding triggers like spicy and greasy food and certain odours can be useful to prevent your nausea from worsening. Brushing your teeth after eating can help. There are safe and effective anti-nausea medications available to treat your symptoms as well. Acupressure wrist bands and ginger may be helpful for some women. There is rarely a concern for the baby's growth in women with nausea and vomiting in early pregnancy unless the mother loses an excessive amount of weight beyond the second trimester. On the contrary, studies have shown that women who experience nausea and vomiting in pregnancy have a lower miscarriage rate compared to women without these symptoms.

A more severe form of morning sickness is known as hyperemesis gravidarum. In hyperemesis gravidarum, excessive vomiting is complicated by significant weight loss of more than 5 percent of body weight, dehydration and electrolyte imbalances in the body. Signs that suggest that your vomiting is severe include abdominal pain, persistent vomiting, blood in the vomit, infrequent urination, dark-coloured urine, or dizziness upon standing. Women with hyperemesis gravidarum usually require hospitalisation for inpatient monitoring and intravenous fluids.

Is my vaginal discharge normal in pregnancy?

In response to hormonal changes and the changes to the pH of the vagina, pregnant women often develop increased vaginal discharge. This discharge is usually thick, white and odourless. While in most instances such discharge is considered normal, it may also be the result of a vaginal infection such as vaginal yeast infection or bacterial vaginosis. Rarely, clear watery discharge may be a presentation of something serious like premature prelabour rupture of membranes (PPROM).

Pregnancy is a risk factor for developing vaginal yeast infection and the fungus *Candida albicans* can be identified by culture from the vagina of one in four pregnant women. Treatment is required only if you suffer symptoms including extreme itchiness, redness and soreness of the vulva and vagina, burning pain during urinating, discomfort during sex and a thick white discharge with a 'cottage cheese' appearance.

Another common cause of vaginal discharge is bacterial vaginosis, where there is an overgrowth of certain bacteria resulting in maldistribution of the normal vaginal flora. The normal vaginal microbiome is disrupted when the numbers of lactobacilli are decreased and species such as *Gardnerella vaginalis* are overrepresented. Women with bacterial vaginosis may complain of a fishy-smelling, grey white discharge that is more pronounced after sexual intercourse. Bacterial vaginosis can be confirmed by taking a vaginal swab and looking for the presence of bacterial vaginosis–related bacteria. Bacterial vaginosis in pregnancy is associated with an increased risk of preterm birth. Treatment can be in the form of oral medication or vaginal pessaries.

Your baby is surrounded by amniotic fluid or 'waters' contained within a membrane bag known as the amniotic sac. Rupture of this amniotic sac resulting in leakage of amniotic fluid before labour at term is normal, however in approximately 3 percent of pregnant women this leakage can happen prematurely. Women presenting with PPROM may feel a trickle or gush of clear fluid, that may be difficult to differentiate from urine. PPROM is a serious complication as the break in the protective membrane layer can lead to infection and preterm delivery.

Is water retention normal in pregnancy?

Increased water retention is a normal physiological change in pregnancy. Close to your due date, the water content from your baby, placenta and amniotic fluid will amount to approximately 3.5 litres. Adding the accumulation as a result of the increase in blood volume and the enlarged uterus and breasts, the extra water volume in your body would amount to at least 6 litres. During pregnancy, in response to hormonal changes, the way your body processes sodium also changes. You may find that you can no longer fit into your favourite heels as your ankles and legs become more swollen, especially towards the end of the day. The extra puffiness you feel will peak in the third trimester. Elevating your feet, avoiding prolonged standing, wearing compression stockings and limiting your sodium intake are all ways to help to ease your symptoms.

Although some amount of water retention is inevitable, there are instances when swelling in pregnancy is abnormal. Two important and dangerous pregnancy complications that can present with swelling are preeclampsia and deep venous thrombosis. Women with preeclampsia develop high blood pressure in pregnancy coupled with other symptoms such as protein in the urine, excessive swelling due to fluid accumulation and blurring of vision. Deep vein thrombosis is the formation of clots in the blood vessels of the body and pregnant women are at much higher risk of this condition compared to non-pregnant women. Swelling related to deep vein thrombosis is usually unilateral and associated with other symptoms such as pain, redness, warmth of the affected leg. Both these conditions are uncommon but can be fatal, so seeking medical treatment early is important.

How much weight should I gain in pregnancy?

The total weight gain recommended during pregnancy is dependent upon your pre-pregnancy body mass index (BMI), as shown in the table below. BMI is easily calculated with the formula BMI = kg/m^2 where kg is a person's weight in kilograms and m^2 is their height in metres squared.

Institute of Medicine's Recommended Weight Gain During Pregnancy Guidelines		
Pre-pregnancy weight category	BMI (kg/m^2)	Recommended total weight gain
Underweight	Less than 18.5	12.5–18 kg
Normal weight	18.5–24.9	11.5–16 kg
Overweight	25.0–29.9	7–11.5 kg
Obese	30 and greater	5–9 kg

As your baby grows bigger, your body will increase its energy requirements. However, it is still not advisable that you 'eat for two'. For a woman with a pre-pregnancy weight in the normal range, she can increase her caloric intake in the second trimester by 300 per day and in the third trimester by 450 per day.

It is now well established that the first nine months in a mother's womb can shape a child's development and health across the lifespan. Under or over nutrition, obesity, maternal stress and gestational diabetes mellitus (GDM) are all potential insults that can increase the child's risk of developing chronic metabolic diseases such as diabetes and hypertension in the future. Prioritising healthy eating and preventing excessive weight gain in pregnancy are important early steps in giving your child the best start in life.

How do I manage constipation in pregnancy?

Constipation is a common woe of expectant mothers. Many factors contribute to worsening constipation in pregnancy. The movement of stool through the bowel slows down due to the hormone progesterone and this delay results in stool becoming more solid as more water is being absorbed. Dehydration due to nausea and vomiting in pregnancy, supplementation with iron as well as being less mobile in pregnancy all contribute to constipation as well. Pregnant women with constipation may develop haemorrhoids, which are swollen blood vessels in the rectum. This can be very uncomfortable and may cause pain, itching or bleeding from the back passage. Increasing fluid and fibre intake, exercise and medications such as stool softeners from your doctor can help to alleviate your symptoms.

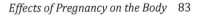

Why are urinary tract infections (UTIs) more common in pregnancy?

The pregnancy hormone progesterone causes relaxation and dilatation of the urinary tract. These changes can result in the reflux of urine from your bladder back up towards your kidneys. The mechanical compression from your enlarging uterus on your bladder can also make it harder for you to let out all the urine and the remaining urine in the bladder becomes a source of infection. There is a risk of ascending infection affecting the kidneys resulting in an increased risk of preterm birth and sepsis. Urinary tract infection in pregnancy must therefore be treated promptly with antibiotics. To prevent getting a urinary tract infection, keep hydrated by drinking a lot of water, wipe yourself from front to back when using the bathroom and empty your bladder shortly before and after sex.

What can I do to ease the pain in my back and joints?

Hormonal changes as well as weight gain in pregnancy result in many changes to your musculoskeletal system. An enlarging uterus and a shift in the centre of gravity results in forward flexion of the neck and lordosis of the back, where the inward curve of the lower back is exaggerated. This altered posture coupled with joint laxity as a result of pregnancy hormones contribute to the development of lower back pain in pregnancy. Wearing low heeled shoes with a good arch support, sleeping on the side with a body pillow or pillow between the knees, sitting in chairs with good support and applying heat, cold or massage to the affected area are a few ways to help with the pain.

The hormone relaxin causes widening and increased mobility of the pelvic joints and the symphysis pubis in preparation for the passage of your baby through the birth canal. Pain at the pelvic joints is called pelvic girdle pain. Women with this condition may complain of pain over the pubic bone, lower back, perineum that worsens with walking up the stairs, getting out of the car or standing on one leg when getting dressed. Avoid prolonged sitting, standing or lifting heavy weights if you have pelvic girdle pain. For back pain and pelvic girdle pain, medication and physiotherapy may be necessary for severe cases.

Pregnant women may also complain of pain or paraesthesia (numbness or a tingling pins and needles feeling) of the hand and wrist because of a condition called carpel tunnel syndrome. This condition occurs when water retention in pregnancy results in excessive pressure on a nerve in your wrist called the median nerve. It is often worse at night and you may even wake up with the feeling of diffuse numbness in your hand. Elevating your arm and keeping your wrist in a neutral position (not flexed) can help to improve symptoms.

How does being pregnant increase my risk of developing venous thrombosis (blood clots)?

Deep vein thrombosis occurs when a blood clot forms in the deep veins of the body, especially the calf or thigh. A part of this clot can break off and travel to the lung, causing a serious condition called pulmonary embolism. During pregnancy, your blood's ability to clot is enhanced as your body's way of preventing excessive blood loss during birth. Decreased mobility and pressure on vessels by your growing womb further adds to this propensity for clotting. Being overweight, having medical conditions such as a history of clotting disorders or lupus, prolonged bed rest during or after your pregnancy, dehydration, long distance travel and having a caesarean section in a previous pregnancy are examples of risk factors that can make your risk of developing deep vein thrombosis in pregnancy higher. Your doctor may start you on compression stockings or an injection called low-molecular-weight heparin as a preventive measure. During your pregnancy, you are encouraged to keep hydrated and to exercise your calf muscles, especially if you are traveling long distances. You should inform your doctor if you develop symptoms suggestive of deep vein thrombosis, such as a painful swollen leg, difficulty breathing or chest pain that worsens when you take a deep breath.

How do I know I am going into labour?

Early in your pregnancy, you may experience painless tightening of your uterus that come and go with no regular pattern. These contractions are known as Braxton Hicks contractions. These contractions tend to occur more frequently as the pregnancy progresses, especially in the last few weeks leading to birth. Studies looking at these contractions found that the electrical activity of the uterus in the early stages of pregnancy are low and uncoordinated, while becoming progressively stronger and synchronised by term. It is almost as if your uterus is preparing itself for the labour process.

It is important to recognise the difference between Braxton Hicks contractions and true labour contractions.

True labour contractions are painful and regular, increasing in severity and frequency. These contractions persist despite changes in position or activity. Another sign of labour is breaking of the water bag. You may feel a gush of clear fluid or a steady trickle dampening your underwear. As part of the labour process, your cervix will stretch and dilate in response to uterine contractions, becoming thinner to allow your baby to pass through the birth canal. As your cervix becomes softer and begins to dilate, the cervical mucus plug is dislodged and you may notice your vaginal discharge containing streaks of mucus with a little fresh blood and this is known as 'show'. All these are signs that you may be going into labour.

Further Reading

ACOG Practice Bulletin No. 189: Nausea and vomiting of pregnancy. *Obstet Gynecol* 2018; 131(1): e15.

American College of Obstetricians and Gynecologists. ACOG Committee opinion no. 548: weight gain during pregnancy. *Obstet Gynecol* 2013 Jan; 121(1): 210–212. doi: 10.1097/01.aog.0000425668.87506.4c. PMID: 23262962.

Piercy CN. *Handbook of Obstetric Medicine* (4th edition) Boca Raton: CRC Press, Taylor & Francis Group (2015).

Franzago M, Fraticelli F, Stuppia L, Vitacolonna E. Nutrigenetics, epigenetics and gestational diabetes: consequences in mother and child. *Epigenetics* 2019; 14(3): 215–235. doi:10.1080/15592294.2019.1582277

Barua S, Junaid MA. Lifestyle, pregnancy and epigenetic effects. *Epigenomics.* 2015; 7(1): 85–102. doi: 10.2217/epi.14.71. PMID: 25687469.

van den Elsen LWJ, Garssen J, Burcelin R, Verhasselt V. Shaping the gut microbiota by breastfeeding: the gateway to allergy prevention? *Front Pediatr* 2019; 7: 47. doi:10.3389/fped.2019.00047

Sheffield JS. *Williams Obstetrics* (24th Edition). New York: McGraw-Hill Education (2014).

Tan EK, Tan EL. Alterations in physiology and anatomy during pregnancy. *Best Pract Res Clin Obstet Gynaecol* 2013 Dec; 27(6): 791–802. doi: 10.1016/j.bpobgyn.2013.08.001. Epub 2013 Sep 4. PMID: 24012425.

Dr Helen Chen

PSYCHOLOGICAL EXPERIENCES AND CHALLENGES IN PREGNANCY AND POSTPARTUM

Take Home Points

1. Emotional care during pregnancy and the postpartum period can help mothers maintain mental wellness during the challenging months of transition into motherhood.
2. Depression and anxiety during pregnancy and in the postpartum period are common, affecting about 1 in 10 women in Singapore.
3. Maternal depression and anxiety can affect child health and development.
4. Interventions are available that can help mothers with depression, this includes medications that are safe in pregnancy and for breastfeeding.
5. Nurturing your bond with baby starts in the womb — talking to your baby can help this process, and you should continue with this as your child grows to build a strong relationship.

Dr Helen Chen is a Senior Consultant Psychiatrist and Head of Department of Psychological Medicine, and is currently practising at the KK Women's and Children's hospital. She is also the Director of the Postnatal Depression Intervention Programme at Duke-National University of Singapore.

"Here comes the stork!"

So, you are planning to have a baby, or perhaps you already have a little bun in the oven? That's delightful! But you've read a little about how rough it can be for some mummies. How one can be floored by morning sickness, or have sleep disrupted by frequent bathroom trips. Or maybe you're already a new mummy, and have been struggling a little to make sense of how your life has utterly changed. Rest assured, you are not alone. The transition to motherhood is truly life-changing, just think of how so many mothers define their lives from the moment they become a mother distinctly from the time before.

Here's a quick snapshot of some of the common conditions that may affect mothers:

Perinatal Depression (also known as Antenatal and Postnatal Depression)

How do I know I have this condition?

If you feel low in mood, are easily tearful or irritable, and have a loss of interest or ability to feel joy/pleasure, have disturbed sleep or poor appetite, difficulty concentrating or feel low in energy, or perhaps even have negative thoughts of self-reproach, hopelessness or suicidal thoughts, you may be depressed. A diagnosis of clinical depression is considered when you have persistent symptoms that last at least two weeks, and they affect your ability to function normally.

Perinatal depression encompasses both antenatal depression as well as postnatal depression. It's particularly hard to tell sometimes as pregnant or postnatal women often feel emotionally sensitive or easily tired, so do look out for the negative thoughts.[1]

Who is at risk?

Perinatal depression often develops because of a combination of factors, so women who are facing multiple challenges, such as marital, work-related stress or have poor social/partner support are more at risk. Those who have experienced past traumatic experiences, especially in their childhood, may also be more vulnerable to having resurfacing difficult emotions, which can lead to the development of perinatal depression. Some personality characteristics can make one more vulnerable, especially those of perfectionism, or high need for control.

Women who have had a past episode of depression, or whose mother or sisters (first degree relatives) have had postnatal depression are also at higher risk of having postnatal depression.

Local studies show that about 1 in 10 women have perinatal depression,[2] whilst 1 in 25 will require clinical attention. The psychological origins of depression may come from issues related to:

i) Loss — for example, loss of one's career goals or ambition
ii) Role transition — for example, from just being a wife, to juggling responsibilities as a mother too
iii) Repressed anger — for example, past childhood trauma or intimate partner abuse.

These inner conflicts can be worked on to help mothers make a successful transition to motherhood.

How can I manage my risk for developing perinatal depression?

Addressing life stresses can help to lessen the likelihood of developing perinatal depression, as each challenge can weigh down on mummy's mood. Being aware of one's source of tension, or stress-points is helpful, so that one can take steps to manage better. For example, it is sometimes hoped that having a baby can improve marital strain, but in fact, a baby can add on to existing problems, given the change in dynamics of the couple's relationship and the additional responsibilities of baby care. Spending quality time on building the marital relationship, or seeking professional help through marital counselling can be important prior to having a baby.

Where possible, try to reduce/avoid getting into situations of high stress, such as changing jobs or moving house before getting pregnant.

Of course, maintaining a healthy lifestyle, having adequate rest and relaxation, good nutrition and exercise or physical activity, as well as having supportive connections are beneficial for good emotional health during childbearing.

How can perinatal depression affect a mummy?

Mummies with perinatal depression not only feel poorly and struggle with the symptoms, but also can find it hard to relate to their babies. This can happen antenatally, so that maternal fetal attachment is impacted, or postnatally with resultant mother-infant bonding difficulties. When mummies are poorly bonded to their babies, it is harder for them to nurture and stimulate their babies well for good development. Sometimes, mummies turn to other ways of coping, such as smoking or drinking, to cope with stress or difficult emotions, and this can be harmful for babies.

Postnatal depression is also linked to early cessation of breastfeeding, as mummies who are struggling with depression often find it hard to have a let-down or to successfully latch their babies.

How is perinatal depression managed?

Perinatal depression can be readily managed with professional help, and chances for recovery is good with early intervention.[4] Supportive counselling or 'talk therapy' can help the mummy make sense of her struggles with the transition to motherhood.[3]

Those with more severe symptoms will benefit from medication that is especially chosen to ensure compatibility with pregnancy and breastfeeding. There are good established guidelines regarding the use of medication for mothers, and with appropriate consideration of risk-benefit ratio, treatment can be safely considered. Addressing any of the other stresses is also important, such as time-off from work, or getting help for marital issues.

What changes should I make to my daily activities if I have perinatal depression?

Be gentle and patient with yourself, allow yourself time to adjust to becoming a mother. Having space for me-time is important, as caring for a baby can be tiring. Try not to take on additional responsibilities, if possible, and be open to receiving help and support from loved ones. Pace yourself in your journey towards motherhood. And most importantly, don't blame yourself as having perinatal depression is not about being weak, or that you are an unloving mother. For if you truly didn't care about your baby, you

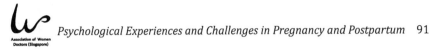

wouldn't be feeling so poorly. And lastly, you don't have to be a perfect mother — you just have to be good enough!

Perinatal Anxiety (also known as Antenatal and Postnatal Anxiety)

How do I know I have this condition?

If you find yourself often troubled by many worries, feeling tense, or having panic attacks, with palpitations, shortness of breath, or tremulousness, you might be suffering from perinatal anxiety.

For some women, anxiety can take the form of feeling a fear of being in crowds (agoraphobia) and they feel particularly anxious about going out on their own. For others, anxiety can take the form of distressing panic attacks (panic disorder) which make them feel as if they are going to collapse or faint and lead to frequent need for medical services. Yet another way anxiety can manifest is in morbid intrusive thoughts, such as thinking they will drop baby, or that baby will stop breathing, or that baby will get sick. Sometimes, the anxiety is soothed by compulsive behaviours such as irrational counting, or excessive checking or washing — this can then develop into a related condition, obsessive compulsive disorder.

Perinatal anxiety encompasses both antenatal anxiety as well as postnatal anxiety. Often, mothers who have depression may also have anxiety features, and vice versa. It's easy to understand why — if you are feeling low and finding it hard to cope normally, you might start to worry about many things, and that can lead to anxiety; or if you are anxious and worried about many things, your spirits will be worn down and that can lead to depression.

Who is at risk?

Just like perinatal depression, perinatal anxiety often develops because of a combination of factors, so women who are facing multiple challenges are more at risk. Those who have past traumatic experiences that have affected their sense of security and confidence, can be more vulnerable.

Anxiety develops in the context of unpredictability and feeling overwhelmed by many stresses. Therefore, in working with mothers, it is important to address these fears and anxieties, to help them make sense of their experience, and regain their sense of calm.

How can I manage my risk for developing perinatal anxiety?

Just like with perinatal depression, addressing life stresses can help to lessen the likelihood of developing perinatal anxiety, as each challenge can weigh down on mummy's sense of calm. Being aware of one's source of tension, or stress-points is helpful, so that one can take steps to manage better. Often, mothers with anxiety have high expectations of themselves, and find it hard to let go and pace themselves.

Maintaining a healthy lifestyle, getting adequate rest and relaxation, having good nutrition and exercise or physical activity, as well as having supportive connections are beneficial for good emotional health during childbearing.

How can perinatal anxiety affect a mummy?

Mummies with perinatal anxiety not only feel poorly and struggle with the symptoms, they also often struggle to bond with their babies. This is because the anxiety is often focused on the infant, so that being with baby makes mum feel tense and wound up. This can lead to mummy avoiding baby, which can impair mother-infant bonding.

Alternatively, some mummies who are anxious can become overprotective and not want anyone else to tend to their babies. This is also not healthy, as over time, little children do need space to grow and develop, and for mummies to let them explore and learn.

Postnatal anxiety is also linked to early cessation of breastfeeding, it can impact a mummy's ability to enjoy breastfeeding especially if she pumps out milk for bottle feeding. She can get caught up in the nitty gritty of pumping and feed volumes, so that it feels as if her primary relationship is with the pump rather than her baby.

How is perinatal anxiety managed?

Just like for perinatal depression, perinatal anxiety can be readily managed with professional help, and chances for recovery is good with early intervention.[4] Supportive counselling, i.e., 'talk therapy', can help the mummy better understand the nature of her worries and her physical symptoms, and allow her to slowly work through her doubts and fears.

Those with more severe symptoms will benefit from medication that is especially chosen to ensure compatibility with pregnancy and breastfeeding.

There are good established guidelines regarding the use of medication for mothers, and with appropriate consideration of risk-benefit ratio, treatment can be safely considered. As previously mentioned, addressing the other stresses is also important, such as taking time off work, or getting help for marital issues.

What changes should I make to my daily activities if I have perinatal anxiety?

Take a step back and allow yourself some time for calming activities. It's ok to not be the best in every aspect of baby's care, and to let your baby lead sometimes in letting you know what he or she needs by crying. For mummies struggling with anxiety, it can be hard to tolerate baby's cries, and the tension mummy feels can be felt by baby, in the way her muscles tighten or how she rocks baby a tad harder. This can make it even harder for baby to settle.

Try any form of mindfulness as this can be beneficial in helping you regain calmness and composure. A good and easy technique to try is to place your hand on your heart, and take three deep and slow calming breaths before you tend to baby. Keep your voice gentle, soft and slow — this can help to calm baby and you!

Pace yourself in your experience with your baby. Often, babies grow and develop so fast and it may seem as if your baby is always one step ahead of your learning. This is normal. Lastly, but very importantly, always remember you don't have to be a perfect mother — you just have to be good enough!

Other Conditions Related to Childbearing

There are also some other less common conditions seen in relation to pregnancy.

Puerperal psychosis

This is a grave condition seen in mothers who are very troubled and for whom there is so much unconscious conflict that it's hard to bring to awareness, so that they present with disturbing symptoms of mood fluctuations, delusional ideas (e.g., of being harmed) and confusion. Because of the risk of harm to self and baby, mothers with puerperal psychosis need urgent medical attention to start medications, and close follow-up. Hospitalisation might be required if there is no means of ensuring the mother's safety, although it can be effective if good quality specialist care with case management is coupled with medication compliance. With prompt treatment, full recovery is possible. As there is a high risk of recurrence in a subsequent pregnancy, mothers with puerperal psychosis are strongly advised to follow up with perinatal mental health specialists for early care planning.

Post-traumatic stress disorder following childbirth

For some mothers, the birthing experience is so traumatic and unpleasant that they develop post-traumatic stress disorder (PTSD) related to childbirth. Some examples include women who needed emergency caesarean section, those who suffer marked tearing of their perineum from natural childbirth, or pelvic fracture. These distressing memories can lead to postnatal depression and/or anxiety and it is important for mothers to talk to someone they trust, or seek professional help, for them to work through their traumatic memories.

Psychological issues related to infertility

The wish to be a mother is natural, and for many women who are unable to conceive, infertility can undermine their sense of womanhood and bring much sadness. With each failed attempt of assisted reproductive intervention, the emotional roller coaster can take its toll on the woman's psyche, and lead to depression. The hormonal treatments needed may also cause mood disturbance, and this can add more strain to the difficult experience.

Being able to find support in her husband gives a woman comfort, and open communication can help a couple cope with the stress of going through infertility intervention. Coming to terms with having infertility helps too — for, after all, womanhood is not just defined by an organ (the womb).

Psychological issues related to pregnancy loss

Any loss of a pregnancy is difficult to cope with, whether intended or otherwise. Women who have had to make the difficult decision to abort an unplanned pregnancy often feel torn and struggle with guilt. Although initially there may be a sense of relief when the crisis of an unwanted pregnancy is resolved with termination, the repressed memories can resurface, especially at times of turmoil. For some women, there can be more psychological disturbance, presenting as post-abortion syndrome, with features of nightmares and flashbacks related to the abortion.

Speaking to a counsellor, and finding a way to forgive oneself can be a step towards healing. It may help to think of how at the point of deciding to go for the abortion, you had made the decision because of the circumstances back then — it wasn't easy and that's why you still carry the guilt through the years.

For those who have lost a much wanted and planned pregnancy, the grief of a miscarriage can be intense and painful — for all the wishes and hopes for a child are lost. Although delivered with good intentions, the oft heard reassurance that, "It's ok, you can try again", can sometimes cause even more hurt — it can feel that the loss was not honoured and given its due period of grieving. Sometimes, a personal gesture of mourning may be helpful for a woman to move on, such as lighting a candle and saying a prayer for the unborn child.

Pseudocyesis

The wish for a child can be so immensely powerful for some women that they might develop pseudocyesis and experience symptoms of pregnancy, like nausea and vomiting, or even missed menstruation. Because the false pregnancy can be carried for several months, it can be very distressing for the woman to be told she is not pregnant. With psychological support and empathic care, the woman with pseudocyesis can gradually come to terms with the reality, and accept her disappointment.

Denial of pregnancy

In some women, pregnancy is not only unwanted, but rejected consciously or unconsciously. This may lead to concealment of their pregnancy, or an irrational lack of awareness of bodily changes. As a result, when delivery finally occurs, the state of unpreparedness and denial can lead to an intense emotional detachment, known as a dissociative state, that results in actions of poor judgement, like flushing the baby down the toilet bowl or throwing the baby down the rubbish chute. These troubled women need help.

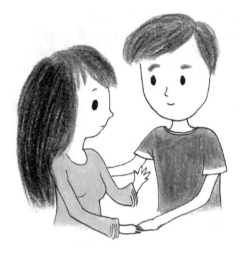

The Good Stuff About Pregnancy and Motherhood

Now that you have learnt all about the various psychological problems that can arise in relation to pregnancy and the postpartum period, you might wonder if childbearing is at all to be embarked upon. Rest assured that the great majority of pregnancies are smooth and uneventful. The motherhood transition is not always smooth, but even in the worst of experiences, mothers have pulled through and shown their strength and courage.

Be honest with your inner feelings, talk about them to a trusted loved one — ideally your partner! Or pen your thoughts in a journal to help you make sense of your worries or doubts. Take good care of your body and mind, and make time for moments of intentional calm that help to foster the practice of mindfulness.

A lovely way to nurture a strong bond with your baby is by **talking to your baby**. You can do this right from the time you are pregnant — did you know your baby can respond to your voice as early as 14 weeks of pregnancy? Keep your voice soft and gentle, and this can help to calm you and also your baby. If you aren't sure what to say, you can try something simple like:

"Good morning baby, how are you today? Mummy's doing ok!"
"It's time for bed, baby, Mummy's going to rest now, I'll talk to you tomorrow!"

And of course, when baby is born, this practice can help to stimulate baby's development as well as nurture your bond. Keep up this easy chat with your baby, as you go about the day, changing diapers, bathing baby or even while feeding.

> *"Here you go, out of this diaper, and soon you will be nice and fresh again!"*
> *"Look what we have here — your favourite romper! We'll keep this away for tomorrow!"*

Just remember that you don't need to be constantly doing this, of course — it would be too tiring! After all, we don't talk to our partners all the time either.

Finally, here's a little sharing from a mother who has pulled through recurrent episodes of puerperal psychosis with her two babies, may it give you hope and reassurance that becoming a loving mother is possible despite having psychological challenges:

> *"To think I used to fear sleeping with her in the same room*
> *— now, we both love waking up to each other."*

References

1. Chen H. Perinatal mental health. In *Textbook of Psychiatry*. Singapore: Institute of Mental Health (2013).
2. Chen H, Tan KH, Chan YH, Lee T. Depressive symptomatology in pregnancy: A Singaporean perspective. *Soc Psy Psych Epid* 2004; 39: 975–979.
3. Ch'ng YC, Wang J, Chen H. Perinatal case management: Caring for our mothers as they care for their babies. *J Paeds Obs Gyn* 2010 Nov/Dec; 227–232.
4. Lee TMY, Bautista D, Chen HY. Understanding how postnatal depression screening and early intervention works in the real world — a Singaporean perspective. *Annals Academy of Medicine Singapore* 2016 Oct; 45(1).

BREASTFEEDING

Take Home Points

1. Establishing a good latch marks the beginning of a successful breastfeeding journey.
2. It is normal for babies to feed frequently, as often as every 30 minutes, during a growth spurt.
3. Most foods and over-the-counter medications are safe for you and your baby during breastfeeding, no need to restrict yourself unnecessarily!
4. Seek help from a breastfeeding counsellor or lactation consultant early to have a more enjoyable journey. You do not have to exhaust your options before seeking help.
5. You own your breastfeeding journey with your baby, ignore naysayers who give non-constructive advice.

Am I making enough milk? How can I increase my milk supply?

These are the 2 most common questions new mothers ask. In the recent decade, breastmilk has been well promoted as a good source of nutrition for

---

Dr Angela Tan is a Family Physician, specializing in home care, palliative care and sexual wellness, and provides island wide home care services.

our babies, with various benefits such as increasing IQ points and building the immune system. Aggressive marketing of formula milk has also been tamed, resulting in more mothers wanting to provide breastmilk for their babies. However, due to high usage of milk substitutes for the last few generations, many new mothers find themselves unable to tap on their own mothers for breastfeeding advice and end up struggling with the whole breastfeeding process. A common belief is that breastfeeding is instinctive, like eating and drinking, but it can be a challenging experience for the new family, as both mother and baby need to learn how breastfeeding actually works. There is a misconception that breastfeeding is only successful if milk flows readily from the breast. However, this is definitely untrue for the majority of new mothers. Without timely troubleshooting from people who actually know about breastfeeding, many assume that they are failing at breastfeeding due to inadequate milk supply.

Studies have shown that it is more common for mothers to perceive they have insufficient milk than for them to actually have insufficient milk. Milk substitutes introduced can contribute to the eventual decline in milk production, ironically making the initial claim true. For a start, let's explore the common myths that make a mother think she has insufficient milk.

Myths of not having enough milk

1. My baby cries after feeding
   Babies cry when they are hungry, but they also cry about any other thing! These include: soiled diapers, colic, when they are sleepy or simply when they are removed from their mothers, aka their 'safety zone'. Some detective work would be great before we attribute all crying to the baby having 'not enough milk'.

2. My baby takes a bottle after feeding
   Young babies take time to learn the concept of 'full'. Most babies will still take liquid from a bottle even when full. Supplementing when not required via bottle feeding interferes with the establishment of breastfeeding.

3. My baby has frequent feeds/ takes a long time to feed
   Babies have small stomachs and breastmilk is really digestible; hence, we are looking at 10–12 feeds per day minimally. Cluster feeding is also

common during a growth spurt (with the first one occurring at the 4–6 week mark) where they will seem to be feeding continuously for hours in a row! Imagine having to limit yourself to drinking water only at 3-hour intervals when you are hungry, the feeling is awful even for adults. Furthermore, some babies feed faster, some slower, just like how we all eat at different speeds. There is no right or wrong way in breastfeeding, it is entirely personal. As such, feeding on cue is the way to go. Formula fed babies may appear to 'last' longer between feeds as formula milk is less digestible than breastmilk (which is also the reason why formula fed babies tend to be constipated), but it definitely does not mean they are 'fuller' or 'better fed'.

4. My baby does not sleep through the night
   Adults do not sleep through the night either. We wake up a few times a night but are able to fall back to sleep on our own without fuss, but babies cannot yet do so. For this reason, sleeping through the night has become a milestone for parents: 'My baby has matured, he/she is well trained'. In actual fact, if a 10-day old baby actually sleeps through the night, it might well be due to other reasons: drowsiness from insufficient milk, dehydration or an infection. Furthermore, feeding on cue during the night is important especially in the first weeks to establish milk supply. Prolactin, a hormone that promotes milk production is more concentrated at night, hence there is more milk at night. When a new mother empties her breasts by feeding her baby at night, it signals to her brain to produce more prolactin and thereby increases overall milk production. In summary, always follow your baby's cue in breastfeeding.

5. My breasts feel soft
   It simply means that your milk supply is getting regulated and thus your breasts are not getting engorged as easily as before; you are doing well Mummy!

6. There is no/ hardly any milk when I pump
   Pumping using a device does not indicate how much milk your baby actually drinks. Breasts are generally less sensitive to a pump than an efficient baby's suckling. Different pumps also have different effects on individual mothers. Focus on the milk transfer when baby is latching rather than the pump output.

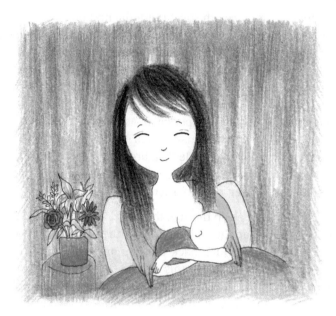

The key to successful breastfeeding is therefore to establish a good latch for efficient milk transfer. However, in the event that responsive breastfeeding is not possible, for example, if the baby is in the ICU, methods to express breastmilk (e.g., hand expression, using an electrical breast pump etc) can be advised by lactation consultants in all our local hospitals.

For the majority of healthy mummies and babies, starting early will increase the chances of success. Take time to attend breastfeeding classes prior to delivery to familiarise yourself with the process and know-hows. Breastfeeding is a learnt skillset for both you and the baby, early preparation helps!

Early skin to skin contact (bare skin) right after birth helps promote baby's rooting instincts and mummy's milk production. ***Let your gynaecologist know you would like skin to skin contact right after birth, there's no real need to bathe your baby immediately.*** The waxy coating (vernix) on a new born has a protective function, keep it on your baby for as long as you can.

Timely troubleshooting in the early days will be crucial in keeping you on the breastfeeding journey. Improper latch, cracked or sore nipples, and a slow let-down reflex are common teething problems many mothers face.

Having a professional on board (lactation consultant, breastfeeding counsellor, doula etc) is highly recommended. Have their numbers and working hours readily accessible so you can reach out to them easily.

Lastly, ensuring that you are well hydrated, eating nourishing food and having good rest are all important factors for adequate milk production and will also give you the energy to care for your baby. Stress can inhibit the let-down reflex, thus preventing milk that is produced from being released. In contrast, relaxation and close bonding with your baby promotes the release of the hormone oxytocin, which triggers the let-down reflex to release the milk in the milk ducts. Good household support is thus crucial to help you settle into your new phase of life as a mother.

Back to the main question, how do we tell baby is actually having enough milk if we can't measure how much they are drinking then? Amount and frequency of poo and pee become our guiding parameters. Gradual weight gain and appropriate milestone development over longer periods of time are also clues. Refer to the infographic below for poo and pee guidelines.

Of course, knowing what is a good latch and seeing/hearing your baby swallow will help reassure you of good milk transfer. The videos here provide a good reference: https://ibconline.ca/breastfeeding-videos-english/

Is my milk safe if I ...?

As breastfeeding mothers, being the sole providers of nutrition for our little ones, we want to make sure what we provide is the best. Hence, it is common for mothers to question if our breastmilk of highest quality and free of 'poisonous' elements at all times. Unfortunately, myths and inappropriate advice from various people (including healthcare professionals) have triggered fears in some new mothers. I hope this section will address most, if not all, of your possible concerns.

1. ... consume any medications?
    Rule of thumb, if the drug in question is commonly prescribed for infants, it is safe for breastfeeding. If it is prescribed during pregnancy, it is also highly likely to be safe. Hence, most commonly prescribed drugs, like paracetamol, flu tablets, antibiotics, do not pose a problem. Radioactive treatment or chemotherapy is of course a very different story altogether. For our understanding, drugs that are ingested orally

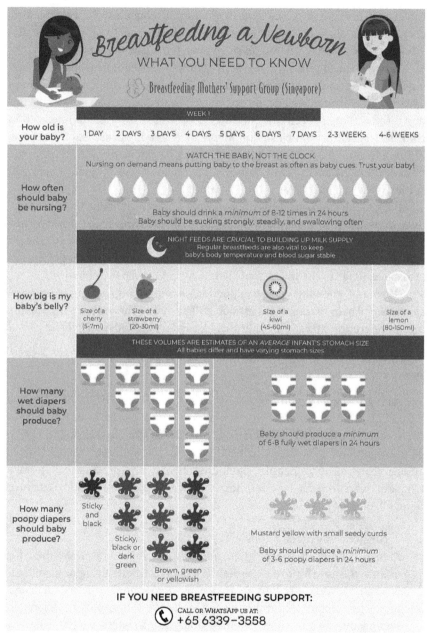

Breastfeeding a Newborn
WHAT YOU NEED TO KNOW
Breastfeeding Mothers' Support Group (Singapore)

	WEEK 1							
How old is your baby?	1 DAY	2 DAYS	3 DAYS	4 DAYS	5 DAYS	6 DAYS	7 DAYS	2-3 WEEKS	4-6 WEEKS

WATCH THE BABY, NOT THE CLOCK
Nursing on demand means putting baby to the breast as often as baby cues. Trust your baby!

How often should baby be nursing?

Baby should drink a *minimum* of 8-12 times in 24 hours
Baby should be sucking strongly, steadily, and swallowing often

NIGHT FEEDS ARE *CRUCIAL* TO BUILDING UP MILK SUPPLY
Regular breastfeeds are also vital to keep
baby's body temperature and blood sugar stable

How big is my baby's belly?

Size of a cherry (5-7ml) · Size of a strawberry (20-30ml) · Size of a kiwi (45-60ml) · Size of a lemon (80-150ml)

THESE VOLUMES ARE ESTIMATES OF AN *AVERAGE* INFANT'S STOMACH SIZE
All babies differ and have varying stomach sizes

How many wet diapers should baby produce?

Baby should produce a *minimum* of 6-8 fully wet diapers in 24 hours

How many poopy diapers should baby produce?

Sticky and black · Sticky, black or dark green · Brown, green or yellowish · Mustard yellow with small seedy curds

Baby should produce a *minimum* of 3-6 poopy diapers in 24 hours

IF YOU NEED BREASTFEEDING SUPPORT:
CALL OR WHATSAPP US AT:
+65 6339-3558

are broken down in our digestive tract, thus only a small amount gets into the bloodstream. From this small amount, only a minute amount actually goes into breastmilk, hence, most of the medications we take do not have much effect on our babies. Breastfeeding mothers, when you are asked to 'pump and dump', it would be good to question the advice. I find http://www.e-lactancia.org/ a very good resource to verify if a drug you have been prescribed is safe for breastfeeding.

2.   ... consume alcohol?
Research shows that approximately 2 percent of ingested alcohol is transferred to milk and this peaks at around 30 minutes to 1 hour after ingestion. It is highly recommended for breastfeeding mothers to not have more than 0.5g of alcohol per kg of body weight. So, for average women, we are looking at 1–2 drinks per day. Some of us who are more cautious, might want to wait for about 2 hours before feeding our babies. There is no need to 'pump and dump', as when the alcohol leaves the blood system, it also leaves the breastmilk. Hence, it is definitely safe for mummies to have a drink and wind down once in a while!

3.   ... consume coffee?
For coffee addicts, caffeine is essential! After all, most mothers of newborns will struggle with insufficient sleep. Studies suggest up to 300 mg of caffeine per day (2–3 cups) has minimal effect on the baby. Nevertheless, some newborns are more sensitive to caffeine exposure and may become fussier and have difficulty falling asleep. In such cases, decaffeinated beverages could be the solution.

4.   ... do my nails, dye my hair, get skin rejuvenation therapy, tattoo my eyebrows?
Topical applications rarely get into breastmilk, so do not worry unduly about pampering yourself in the midst of all the busyness of having a new baby.

How can I store my milk safely?

This infographic says it all!

Association of Women
Doctors (Singapore)

STORING EXPRESSED BREAST MILK (UPDATED 2019)

Breastfeeding
Mothers'
Support Group

Recommendations here are suitable for
- healthy term babies (follow doctor's instructions for warded/preterm babies)
- typical climate conditions in Singapore and similar tropical countries

CHEST FREEZER/DEEP FREEZER
(temps between -20°C to -10°C)
Frozen milk is best before 6 months but lasts
longer in good freezers. The taste of frozen
milk tends to decline after 3 months.

UP TO
12
MONTHS

SELF-CONTAINED FREEZER UNIT
(temps between -10°C to 0°C)
Keep milk well-sealed and at the back of the
freezer away from door. Milk should be frozen
immediately once expressed for best results.

UP TO
6
MONTHS

REFRIGERATOR COMPARTMENT
(temps between 0°C to 4°C)
Freshly expressed milk is best before 3 days,
but can last up to 8 days at the coldest part of
the fridge, away from the door.

UP TO
8
DAYS

COOLER WITH ICE PACKS
(temp of approximately 15°C)
Surround milk with ice packs and keep lid
closed as much as possible.

UP TO
24
HOURS

AIR-CONDITIONED ROOM
(temps between 16°C to 26°C)
Milk is best before 4 hours but can last longer
at low temperatures. However, chill milk ASAP
if not being consumed immediately.

UP TO
8
HOURS

ROOM TEMPERATURE
(temps between 28°C to 35°C)
Milk should be placed in a cool area out of
direct sunlight, but chill milk ASAP if not
being consumed immediately.

UP TO
3
HOURS

UNTOUCHED WARMED MILK
(temp of approximately 37°C)
Milk should be returned to the fridge within
an hour and can be used for the next feed
within 3 hours.

UP TO
1
HOUR

★ ALWAYS SMELL AND TASTE MILK TO VERIFY FRESHNESS
- breast milk should never be sour or rancid
- leftover milk that has touched saliva is generally safe for
  another feed if refrigerated and served within 1-2 hours
- as long as the breast milk is drinkable, it is still superior
  to formula milk

- Eglash, A, & Simon, L. (2017). ABM Clinical Protocol #8 Human Milk Storage Information for Home Use for Full-Term Infants BREASTFEEDING MEDICINE, 12.7th ser.

IF YOU NEED BREASTFEEDING SUPPORT:
CALL OR WHATSAPP US AT:
+65 6339-3558

My breast hurts, is it a blocked duct? Is it mastitis?

1. Engorgement
    There are some common reasons why some breastfeeding mummies experience pain in their breast(s). In the first few days after delivery, engorgement can happen as the milk starts coming in. Engorgement can happen to both sides of the breasts and cause minor to moderate discomfort. It can worsen if milk is not effectively removed from the breast e.g., due to a poor latch. Treatment is focused on effective milk removal. Do consult a lactation consultant to assess your baby's latch if you are not sure. Cold cabbage leaves applied to the breast is a common home remedy that seems to work well for many. However, be mindful it may reduce your milk supply if overused.

2. Blocked duct
    A blocked duct happens when milk is not flowing well through a particular milk duct or it is completely blocked, resulting in a painful lump or wedge-shaped engorgement on the breast. Some redness is present around the area and the lump is warm and painful to touch. Mild fever may also be present. A blocked milk duct can be triggered by a milk bleb/ blister on the nipple which prevents milk from being released from a particular segment of the breast. It can also be triggered when milk is inadequately removed from the breast because of poor latch, dragging out of feeding/pumping times, over supply etc. The main treatment is to ensure efficient milk transfer every 2 hours or so, for milk to be removed from the clogged area(s). Do so by latching the baby and coupled this with breast compression. Position the baby so that his/her chin points towards the blocked area, this will enhance the unclogging process. With nursing, the lump usually decreases in size and becomes less painful even if not fully resolved. Heat compressions and gentle massages can help in mild situations. However, if the blockage is severe and shows no improvement after a day or 2, it is best to seek professional help, such as from a lactation consultant, before mastitis ensues.

    In multicultural Singapore, it is also common for mothers to seek help from traditional masseuses or physicians of traditional medicine. It is important to make sure these individuals are professionals, as there have been cases of mild blockage being escalated to abscess due to inappropriate management. Do check out past reviews/testimonials of who you are about to hire. Blocked ducts do not require the use of antibiotics for treatment.

For mothers with recurrent blocked ducts, it is important to examine and resolve the triggers. A previous blocked duct or mastitis that was inadequately treated is a major risk factor. Poor latch, constrictive clothing (e.g., underwire bra or tight-fitting clothes) or positioning that puts prolonged pressure on the breast can result in poor milk drainage. Stress and being overtired can definitely cause poor milk drainage too.

Mothers with recurrent blocked ducts can also consider taking daily lecithin supplements to help reduce the viscosity (stickiness) of their breastmilk and hence reduce the likelihood of blockages. Lecithin helps to increase the percentage of polyunsaturated fatty acids in the milk and in no way changes the nutrition value of your breastmilk nor does it have side effects for yourself or baby.

3. Milk blister/bleb
    Should there be a milk blister/bleb, popping it with a sterile needle and allowing the milk to flow out will ease the blockage. This is can be done by a lactation consultant if you are not comfortable doing so yourself. A milk blister/bleb can be very painful and hence latching the baby seems very counterintuitive. However, it is important to keep latching to clear the blocked areas. Apply nipple cream generously after each feed to promote recovery of the nipple. Prior to feeding, you can also squeeze some breastmilk out and apply it over the affected nipple as a moisturiser to reduce the pain. With a correct latch, the pain usually eases after the initial latch.

    Should you be getting recurring milk blisters/blebs, it is important to reassess the latch as a poor latch is a common cause for nipple injury causing the formation of milk blister/bleb. A baby with a seemingly okay latch initially may develop a poor latch over time possibly due to the presence of a subtle tongue-tie that was not picked up in the early days. There are some lactation consultants and paediatricians who are more experienced in picking up tongue-ties if you are not sure of whether your baby has one.

4. Mastitis
    Mastitis refers to the inflammation of the breast, it can be caused by obstruction e.g., a blocked milk duct, an infection or allergy. Symptoms are similar to a blocked duct but are usually more intense, and there is fever (>38.5 degrees Celsius), chills and rigors. If the obstruction is

relieved early and symptoms improve within 12–24 hours, antibiotics may not be necessary. However, if symptoms do not improve or get worse within 12-24 hours, it is advised to start oral antibiotics (in Singapore, Augmentin is commonly prescribed).

To summarise, treatment of blocked ducts and mastitis include the following: heat, massage, rest, and emptying the breast. These may cause a temporary reduction in milk supply. Continual and regular nursing/pumping will help bring the milk supply back up.

5. Breast abscess

If left untreated or inadequately treated, a bacterial mastitis can progress to an abscess which is more challenging to treat. An abscess consists of a pocket of pus in the infected area. Simple aspiration with needle and syringe can be done for small abscesses. Large ones may require drainage under the guidance of ultrasound machines. If continuing breastfeeding is important for you, find a breastfeeding friendly surgeon to help you best manage the abscess. Surgical options are less favourable nowadays due to a prolonged time of healing and breastfeeding can be disrupted due to hospital stay. That said, breastfeeding can be continued in the presence of breast abscess.

Should I latch or pump exclusively?

A good number of mothers who are pumping exclusively started their breastfeeding journey not knowing what to expect. The start of the breastfeeding journey can be defined as traumatic to some mothers as there is so much uncertainty around it especially when we cannot tell how much milk the baby has drunk. Are we starving our babies? Why is baby still crying? Why is the baby screaming every time I put her on my breast? The stabbing pain with every latch on your sore nipples is certainly unnerving. Not forgetting the sleepless days and nights to try and make it all work. Hence, some mothers decide to start their pumping journey early, particularly if latching seems almost impossible for them; it is also much more comforting to be able to visualise how much their babies have drunk.

Over time however, mothers who are able to latch their babies directly have an 'easier' life than mothers who pump. Mothers who pump have to manage the breast pump and its multiple parts — washing and sterilising the pump parts and milk bottles, storing the milk, and warming up the milk. During breastfeeding, we get to enjoy time bonding with our babies, but pumping takes at least 30–60 minutes each time, and this is time away from our babies. The breast pump is also known to drain milk less effectively than a baby's suckle, thereby increasing the chance of blocked ducts/mastitis.

Some mothers who start off being exclusive pumpers are able to train themselves and their babies to latch again months later. Others remain exclusive pumpers throughout their breastmilk provision journey.

Other than the steep learning curve of breastfeeding in the initial stages, unhelpful comments from people around us can deter us from breastfeeding exclusively. For instance, a common one is that your baby is using you as a pacifier. This often triggers a fear of being manipulated by our babies which lead us to forget that breastfeeding is how nature intended for us to nurture our little ones. As mentioned above, babies need the breast regularly for water, nutrition and comfort; how is that manipulation? It is a fact that pacifiers were invented to substitute breasts, not the other way around.

On this breastfeeding journey, it is important to trust your own instinct as a mother and ask for plenty of support right from the start to get you through. You are never alone. Of course, there are mothers who sail through the breastfeeding journey and never once experience a blocked duct or sore nipple. Remember though that we are all unique individuals with our own journeys, so don't compare. Do what is best for you and your baby. And yes, if pumping is what works for you due to various reasons, go for it. It can be more challenging in some aspects, but it is still an expression of love for your baby.

I am going back to work, what should I do?

The first question to ask yourself is 'what are my breastfeeding goals?' Most mothers in our local setting end their maternity leave after 4 months, a time when babies are still very dependent on milk for nutrition. Is it your goal to breastfeed until your baby is 6 months old (and can start taking some solids) or 1 year old (where milk is still the main source of nutrition) or beyond? It is important to keep pumping while at work in order to maintain supply and to prevent milk stasis which often results in blocked ducts. Mothers who return to work are usually able to maintain their supply by pumping while at work and latching baby while at home.

An increasing number of companies have become more supportive of breastfeeding by providing a room for mothers to express their milk and allowing them to pump during office hours. If your company is not quite supportive, do speak to your manager/supervisor to see if an arrangement can be made. There are also a number of handsfree electric pumps available commercially, where you can express milk while working at your desk. If you have any challenges in expressing milk at work, feel free to touch base with the Breastfeeding Mothers Support Group (BMSG) Singapore. This organisation has regular workshops to share about various breastfeeding-related topics and provides platforms where you can ask other mothers in similar situations how they overcome their challenges.

For mothers who exclusively breastfeed their babies while on maternity leave, the common question is, when do I need to start freezing my milk? Fret not, you only need to start 1 week in advance. Mothers who breastfeed exclusively often adjust well to their babies' needs, hence they rarely have too much extra after a feed to pump out. Therefore, the best way is to collect milk while nursing your baby. A silicone milk collector such as the Haakaa pump helps collect let-down milk from one breast while your baby feeds from the other. There might not be a lot at each collection, perhaps 20mls, perhaps 60mls. It doesn't matter, store whatever amount you can collect in the fridge, and when you reach the desired amount (the amount you want to freeze per feed, e.g., 120mls), combine everything into a milk storage bag and freeze it. Within a week, most mothers will be able to collect 4–8 packets of 120mls frozen milk for use on Day 1 of them going back to work. After which, whatever you pump during the day at work will be for your baby's intake the next day. Hence, there is no need to stress yourself to get prepared too early nor to spend too much time pumping nothing at your desk. Spend precious time with your little one before you head back to work!

What if my baby only wants to drink from the breast?

There are some babies who hold extremely high standards as to how milk is delivered to their mouths. These babies stress their mothers and caregivers intensely in the initial stages as they refuse artificial breasts (aka milk bottles) and will only drink from the breast. They scream and wail as though they are to be fed with poison when a milk bottle is put to their mouths. If you happen to have a baby as such, well, take heart, he/she feels that you are not replaceable!

What can you do then? Sometimes changing bottles and trying different teats help. Sometimes, feeding them when they are half asleep (known as dream feeding) helps. Sometimes, using a cup or a spoon helps. Be patient, try different things. You will be able to find a good number of creative methods that other mothers have shared on social media groups like the BMSG Facebook group. And if nothing seems to work even after some weeks, your baby may well have decided to do reverse cycling instead. This means they will drink more frequently at night to make up for what they didn't get in the day. Co-sleeping and side-latching will be helpful to help you get your desired sleep while your baby helps herself/ himself to your milk buffet.

It will thus be important to reassure caregivers that it is ok when your baby refuses the bottle, and to encourage them to try other methods. Also, no matter how small an amount baby takes, it is good enough. Remember, the survival instincts in your baby will ensure he/she doesn't starve himself/ herself. Your baby will still take sips throughout the day to ensure hydration. And you will be surprised how well babies can adapt, continuing to play and sleep as usual. Once you have hit the 6-month milestone, solids can be gradually introduced, then there will be even less to worry about. So, hang in there!

How do I wean off breastfeeding?

Weaning off breastfeeding is a very personal choice; it will be good not to let society or other people force you into it. In other word, disregard comments like, "breastmilk is no longer nutritious after the first 6 months", "you shouldn't let your baby control your life", "isn't it shameful for your 2-year-old to still be breastfeeding", "breastfeeding will prevent you from having another baby", etc. All these statements are not true. Breastmilk remains nutritious even in toddlerhood and is a good source of vitamins and antibodies, no matter how long we have been breastfeeding. It also builds and maintains mother-child bonding. And it can be a lifesaver when your little one is sick and refuses all oral intake of other liquids or solids. At this time, cuddling up to mummy and suckling at the breast is all that they need to feel better.

When getting ready to wean, ask yourself these questions: Have I reached my breastfeeding goals? Am I ready? Is my baby ready? If the answer to all 3 questions is yes, you are good to go. To prevent milk stasis and blocked ducts, it is important to gradually drag out your pumping frequency or nursing frequency, so that your breasts adjust to the decline in supply. There are also herbs/tea (e.g., Sage tea) that can help reduce milk supply. Applying cold cabbage leaves can help relieve engorgement if it happens.

If for any medical or personal reasons, you need to stop breastfeeding abruptly, speak to your family doctor to see if medications (e.g., Dostinex) will be suitable for you.

Another common question is: Do I need to wean if I am pregnant? The simple answer is no, breastfeeding is safe for normal pregnancies. For mummies with a high risk of pre-term labour and/or miscarriage, breastfeeding might not be advisable, but check with your doctor. A dip in your milk supply might happen in the 2nd trimester or a change in the taste of the breastmilk due to colostrum production might prompt your baby to self-wean. However, some babies continue to nurse as usual. Some mummies might experience breastfeeding aversion and agitation that makes breastfeeding immensely uncomfortable and hence they choose to wean. If you would like to continue breastfeeding whilst pregnant, self-care is important. Ensure you have enough rest and nutrition to cope with caring for your older child and being pregnant.

I hope this chapter has answered most of the nagging issues and uncertainty around breastfeeding. Remember, you are not alone in this motherhood journey ... do reach out when you need help/advice.

These are some helpful resources for further reading:

1. Breastfeeding Mothers' Support Group, Singapore, https://breastfeeding.org.sg/
2. https://kellymom.com/
3. https://ibconline.ca/

COMMON GYNAECOLOGICAL CONDITIONS

Take Home Points

1. Fibroids, endometriosis, cysts and polycystic ovaries are common gynaecological problems which can also affect fertility.
2. See a gynaecologist if your periods are irregular, heavy or painful.
3. Maintain a healthy diet and lifestyle to minimise menstrual and gynaecological problems.
4. Different treatment options are available depending on your symptoms, age, desire for fertility, and risks for cancer.
5. If surgery is needed, laparoscopic or minimally invasive surgery may be possible and will usually allow a faster recovery compared with abdominal surgery.
6. Start planning for a family as early as possible — women are born with a fixed number of eggs in the ovaries, and our egg count as well as egg quality will decline as we get older.

(Continued)

Dr Kelly Loi is an Obstetrician and Gynaecologist, specializing in Fertility, Reproductive Medicine and Surgery, and is the Medical director of Health & Fertility Centre for Women at Mount Elizabeth Medical Centre, and Mount Elizabeth Hospital Fertility Centre.

(*Continued*)

7. Seek fertility treatment early if needed — as our egg reserve drops, the success rates with fertility treatment will decrease, and our miscarriage risks will rise with increasing age.
8. Fertility problems can also be due to male factor issues, so encourage your partner to be tested too.
9. Maintain a healthy diet and lifestyle to protect and improve your fertility.
10. Do not despair if difficulty is encountered as there are different fertility treatment options for different couples.

Fibroids

What are fibroids?

Uterine fibroids or leiomyomata are smooth muscle cell tumours of the uterus. They are the most common type of benign gynaecologic tumours in women of reproductive age.

While the exact cause of fibroids is unknown, they are linked to high levels of oestrogen. The female hormone oestrogen appears to promote their growth. This is why a high proportion — about one-third — of women get them in their peak reproductive years. They typically get larger over time until menopause and then shrink with falling levels of oestrogen.

Am I at risk of having fibroids?

The lifetime prevalence is around 30 percent.

Some factors that are associated with an increased risk of fibroids include:

- Family history: women whose mothers and sisters have fibroids are more likely to have them too
- No previous pregnancies
- Obesity
- Vitamin D deficiency.

What symptoms can fibroids cause?

Symptoms depend on the size and location of fibroids. Fibroids can vary in size, ranging from tiny 'seedlings' that are undetectable by visual examination to large masses that enlarge and distort the uterus. In many cases, they do not often cause overt symptoms. However, excessively large or numerous fibroids can cause prolonged, heavy and/or painful periods.

Large fibroids can also affect surrounding organs and cause pressure effects. Those that grow on the front wall of the uterus near the bladder may cause urinary symptoms, such as urgency and frequency or urinary retention. Other common symptoms of uterine fibroids include pelvic pressure or pain, constipation, backache or leg pains.

How are fibroids diagnosed?

Pelvic examination: A physical examination may indicate the presence of fibroids. During a pelvic exam, the doctor palpates (manually feels) areas in your pelvis for abnormalities, such as cysts on your reproductive organs or adhesions (scar tissue) behind your uterus. However it is often not possible to feel small fibroids. So the doctor's second step is an ultrasound scan.

Ultrasound scan: An ultrasound scan is used to detect fibroids. An ultrasound is a painless, non-invasive procedure that uses sound waves to obtain a 'picture' of the uterus. To capture the images, a device called a transducer is either pressed against the abdomen or inserted into the vagina (transvaginal ultrasound).

If heavy menstrual bleeding is a concern with fibroids, blood tests may be ordered to determine your iron levels and rule out other bleeding disorders or thyroid problems.

While there is a very low chance (around 0.5 percent) of a fibroid turning cancerous, women should undergo regular scans every 6 to 12 months to detect any abnormities.

Will fibroids affect my fertility?

Many women with fibroids have successful pregnancies. However, depending on the size or location of the fibroid, fertility and pregnancy may be affected.

Fertility may be affected by large fibroids which distort the cavity of the womb, or those which grow into the cavity of the womb, also known as submucosal fibroids. It is well established that submucosal fibroids have a negative impact on fertility and pregnancy.

Submucosal fibroids may block a fallopian tube or the entrance to the uterus, making it harder for eggs and sperm to meet. Submucosal fibroids or large fibroids which affect the cavity of womb may also prevent a fertilised egg from attaching itself to the lining of the womb. This may cause miscarriages.

Hence, an important aspect in evaluating fibroids is to determine if the fibroid is submucosal, and the degree to which it impinges on the cavity of the womb or endometrium.

Will fibroids affect my pregnancy?

During pregnancy, around one third of fibroids may decrease in size, one third remain the same but one third may increase in size. Depending on size and location, fibroids may affect the position of the baby and cause problems during labour and delivery. In some cases, a Caesarean section may be required.

Another problem that may affect patients with large fibroids in pregnancy is pain. The pain can be so severe that some patients have required hospitalisation for bed rest and pain relief.

How are fibroids treated?

The decision on the best treatment option for fibroids depends on a variety of factors. These include:

- Size of the fibroids and the symptoms caused e.g., severity of pain
- Desire for fertility
- Risk for cancerous changes.

Observation:
For fibroids which are small — less than 5cm in diameter, and for women who do not face significant symptoms, conservative management may be sufficient. This includes observation with regular ultrasound scans to check that they remain stable.

Medication:

Drugs may be prescribed to relieve symptoms such as heavy or painful menstruation.

Surgery:

There are also several surgical options to treat fibroids. A myomectomy may be used to remove uterine fibroids while leaving the uterus in place. Though the fibroids are removed, new uterine fibroids may take their place over time, so this procedure is better for women who still plan to have children.

For women with numerous uterine fibroids and who have passed their childbearing years, a hysterectomy may be recommended. This surgery involves removing the entire uterus and all the fibroids.

If surgery is required, transvaginal approach using hysteroscopy may be sufficient for submucous fibroids. For larger fibroids, the surgical approach may be through minimally invasive surgery — also called a laparoscopy. During laparoscopy small incisions are made to allow the use of slender viewing instruments. Alternatively, open surgery — also called a laparotomy may be needed. This will usually involve making a larger cut along the 'bikini line'.

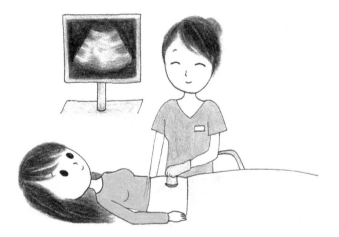

Endometriosis

What is endometriosis?

Endometriosis is a condition in which cells from the endometrium (the lining of the womb) are found outside the womb in the pelvis and around the ovaries and fallopian tubes where they attach and form cysts and lesions. Endometriosis can also take hold almost anywhere on, behind or around the womb: in the peritoneum (the tissue that lines the abdominal wall and surrounds most of the organs in the abdomen), on the bowel and the bladder. It can also develop deep within the muscle wall of the uterus where it is called adenomyosis.

The cause of endometriosis is not known but the most likely explanation is that during menstruation, some of the blood containing cells from the endometrium flows backwards into the pelvic area via the fallopian tubes. Once in the pelvic area, the cells attach themselves to other organs and begin to grow. With each period more cells from the endometrium enter the pelvic area while those already present are stimulated to grow by the hormonal fluctuations of the menstrual cycle.

Am I at risk of getting endometriosis?

Endometriosis affects 10 to 15 percent of women of reproductive age. Factors that increase the risk of endometriosis include:

- Family history: women whose mothers and sisters have endometriosis are more likely to have them too
- Having fewer babies later in life might cause an increase in cases of endometriosis.

What are the symptoms of endometriosis?

Typical symptoms include painful periods, pelvic pain and discomfort or pain during sexual intercourse.

How is it diagnosed?

Pelvic examination: During a pelvic exam, the doctor palpates (manually feels) areas in your pelvis for abnormalities, such as cysts on your reproductive organs or adhesions (scar tissue) behind your uterus. However, it is often not possible to feel small areas of endometriosis unless they have caused a cyst to form.

Ultrasound scan: Ultrasound imaging will not definitively tell the doctor whether endometriosis is present, but it can identify ovarian cysts (endometriomas) and large growths in other areas.

Laparoscopic surgery: To be certain, the patient may need to undergo a laparoscopy to look inside the abdomen for signs of endometriosis. Samples of suspected endometriosis tissue may be taken for biopsy. Laparoscopy can provide information about the location, extent and size of the endometrial growths to help determine the best treatment options.

How does it affect a woman's fertility and pregnancy chances?

Endometriosis can develop on the ovaries where it can form cysts (known as chocolate cysts) as well as in or on the fallopian tubes, causing fertility issues as the growths can block the passage of both sperm and eggs. Endometriosis can also cause an inflammatory environment in the pelvis. Surgery to diagnose and remove endometriosis ovarian cysts can improve fertility.

How is it treated?

Observation:
Simple painkillers may be taken to ease the pelvic pain. However, endometriosis tends to progress over time and regular scans and follow-up consultations will be needed.

Medication:
Several hormonal treatments are available. Contraceptive treatments such as the combined oral contraceptive pills and progestin-only intrauterine devices like Mirena and contraceptive implants are sometimes prescribed for mild to moderate endometriosis. They may reduce or eliminate the pain of endometriosis by helping to control the hormones responsible for the build-up of endometrial tissue each month, thus making periods shorter and lighter.

Another hormone therapy, Visanne, an oral progestin medication, also reduces the production of certain hormones associated with menstruation. Most women find they stop menstruating after taking it for a few months so it is effective at reducing period and pelvic pain. Visanne is a good option for women who need to control their endometriosis but also hope to get pregnant in the future. Visanne is often prescribed after women have had surgery to remove endometriosis to ensure it does not return.

Gonadotropin-releasing hormone (GnRH) agonist injections are also used often after surgery to prevent ovulation, menstruation, and the growth of endometriosis. However, this treatment sends the body into a 'menopausal' state which causes side effects similar to menopause, including hot flashes, tiredness and bone loss. GnRH agonists may be used for several months. As with all hormonal treatments, endometriosis symptoms return after women stop taking GnRH agonists.

Surgery:

For women who hope to get pregnant, conservative surgery to remove as much endometriosis as possible while preserving the uterus and ovaries may be required to increase their chances of success. If the endometriosis is causing severe pain, surgery may also help to relieve it; however, the endometriosis and pain may return unless a hormone treatment like Visanne is used to control it.

These days, surgery is usually done laparoscopically but traditional abdominal surgery may be required for very severe and extensive cases.

If pregnancy is the woman's primary concern, assisted reproductive technologies, such as in vitro fertilisation, might be needed, aside from conservative surgery. Once the woman has had a baby, she can continue to undergo hormonal treatments such as Visanne to manage the endometriosis.

For severe cases of endometriosis where fertility is not a concern, a total hysterectomy and bilateral salphingo-oophorectomy (THBSO) may be required. A THBSO removes the uterus and cervix as well as both ovaries. As one cannot get pregnant after a hysterectomy it is typically considered a last resort for women in their reproductive years.

Ovarian Cysts

What are ovarian cysts?

Ovarian cysts refer to fluid collections in the ovaries. Most ovarian cysts are 'functional cysts' which contain clear fluid. Such cysts are relatively common and occur in relation to the development of the egg in the ovary during the menstrual cycle. The cysts arise when there are problems with ovulation and the egg is not released properly.

Other cystic structures in the ovary which are not parts of the ovulation cycle are called 'pathological ovarian cysts', or 'tumours'. These are often benign or non-cancerous, but they can also be cancerous. Some examples include endometriotic cysts and dermoid cysts. Dermoid cysts may be filled with various types of tissues, including hair and skin. Endometriotic cysts on the other hand contain old blood and endometrial cells shed from the lining of the uterine cavity.

Am I at risk of getting ovarian cysts?

Factors that may increase the risk for developing a functional ovarian cyst include:

- Use of fertility drugs such as clomiphene citrate or other such ovulation induction medication
- Use of low dose progesterone-only contraception such as certain pills, hormone implants, and intra-uterine devices.

What are the symptoms and possible complications?

Depending on the nature and size of the cyst, there may be different symptoms.

Most small functional cysts measuring under 5cm, do not cause symptoms. However, the larger the cyst is, the more likely it is to cause symptoms. These include: irregular menstrual bleeding, or pain in the lower belly, usually in the middle of the menstrual cycle.

Generally, ovarian cysts — especially dermoid cysts — are at risk of ovarian cyst 'accidents'. These include ovarian torsion where the ovary twists around its stalk. When this happens, there is often sudden, severe pain, often with nausea and vomiting. Other times, the cysts may break open (rupture) and bleed. Some ruptured cysts bleed to the extent that treatment is needed to prevent heavy blood loss.

In addition, endometriosis and endometriotic cysts tend to cause recurring and worsening pain with each menstrual period, Endometriotic cysts may also lead to pain during sexual intercourse. These cysts are associated with infertility.

How are ovarian cysts diagnosed?

Pelvic examination and ultrasound scan may help to diagnose the size and nature of the cyst.

Further imaging with CT scans and MRI scans may help to provide more information and assess risks of cancer in the ovarian cyst. Blood tests such as ovarian cancer markers like CA 125 may also be performed to monitor the risk for cancer.

What are the treatment options?

The decision on the best treatment option for ovarian cysts depends on a variety of factors. These include:

- Size of the cyst and the symptoms caused e.g., severity of pain from the ovarian cysts
- Desire for fertility
- Risk for cancerous changes.

Observation:

Functional cysts usually resolve without treatment with time. However, some ovarian cysts may be persistent or increase in size over time. If there are symptoms of pain or risks of cancer, surgery may be necessary. Ultrasound scans are useful for the monitoring of ovarian cysts.

Medication:

Medication such as painkillers may be prescribed for pain from an ovarian cyst. In some cases, hormonal suppression of the menstrual cycle with birth control pills or injections may be recommended.

Surgery:

Surgery may be advisable if the cysts cause symptoms, are persistent and there is a risk of cancerous change. Endometriotic cysts in particular have an adverse effect on fertility and surgery may help increase pregnancy success rates before fertility treatment.

Cystectomy refers to surgery to remove the cysts while leaving the ovary intact. For women who wish to maintain fertility, cystectomy allows the cysts to be removed while conserving the ovaries. Cystectomy will enable the cysts to be sent for biopsy and confirm whether they are cancerous. Such surgery is usually performed by laparoscopy (minimally invasive or keyhole method). If the risk of cancer is high, open or abdominal surgery may be advised to further assess where cancer cells may have spread.

Surgery to remove the ovary, also known as oophorectomy, is the permanent solution for ovarian cysts but the ovary is an important source of hormones. If early menopause occurs, hormone replacement therapy may be needed.

Polycystic Ovary Syndrome

What is polycystic ovary syndrome or PCOS?

Polycystic ovary syndrome (PCOS) is a condition where ovulation (the release of an egg) may not take place as often as normal. On ultrasound scan, many egg follicles which appear as small cysts (small, fluid-filled sacs) are found in the ovaries.

Am I at risk of having PCOS?

PCOS is estimated to affect 5–20 percent of the general female population.

Environmental influences such as nutrition and lifestyle resulting in weight gain further influence the expression of the disease.

What are the symptoms?

The usual symptoms of PCOS result from an imbalance of hormones and you could have higher levels of testosterone than normal. Symptoms may include:

- Irregular menstruation
- Acne and hirsutism
- Obesity
- Cardiovascular disease
- Diabetes.

There is a high incidence of insulin resistance and hyperinsulinaemia and an increase in androgen production.

How is it diagnosed?

Diagnosis requires a detailed medical history and investigations, including:

- Blood tests for female and male hormone levels
- Ultrasound scan.

In view of the higher risks of impaired glucose tolerance and diabetes, other special investigations include:

- 75g oral glucose tolerance test
- Fasting cholesterol, lipids, triglycerides test.

How does PCOS affect fertility and pregnancy?

As a result of hormone imbalance, a PCOS patient may not ovulate regularly, resulting in irregular menstruation and fertility issues.

Once pregnant, patients with PCOS are at an increased risk of miscarriage and developing gestational diabetes mellitus (GDM). They should be screened for abnormal glucose tolerance and GDM in pregnancy.

What are the general treatment strategies?

Maintaining a healthy body mass index through healthy food choices and regular aerobic exercise are important for long term health.

If fertility is not desired, symptomatic treatment should be given as needed.

There is a well-known association between PCOS, endometrial hyperplasia and uterine cancer.

Patients with irregular and infrequent periods should therefore be advised on a regular use of oral hormone treatment to induce menstrual bleeding in a cyclical fashion, on 3–4 monthly basis.

For acne and hirsutism, medical management includes use of combined oral contraceptives. Cosmetic treatments may also help.

If fertility is desired, several options may be considered depending on other fertility factors.

Medications:

Oral fertility drugs such as clomiphene citrate or letrozole may help to induce ovulation. Some side effects include: hot flushes, headache, nausea.

Blood sugar-lowering drugs such as Metformin may be prescribed to improve ovulation response. Some side effects include gastric issues and diarrhoea.

Fertility treatment with IUI or IVF:

IUI (intra-uterine insemination) or IVF (in-vitro fertilisation) may be suitable and more effective for some patients who have other fertility factors. IUI or IVF may also be needed for those who have been found to be resistant to medical treatment, or have not succeeded with fertility drugs alone. In such cases, the hormonal injections given during the IUI or IVF process will usually be effective in inducing ovulation.

Surgery:

Laparoscopic Ovarian Drilling is a surgical technique which may help to induce spontaneous ovulation. Some studies have found up to 60 percent respond with resumption of cycles. Effects are transient up to 1 year for 50 percent of responders and 50 percent conceive within 1 year. However, there are the associated risks of surgery and anesthesia.

Infertility

What is infertility?

Infertility is defined as the inability to conceive after 1 year of trying.

How long does it normally take for couples to conceive? What percentage of couples will be pregnant within the first 6 months of trying? Within the first year?

Around 70 percent of couples will become pregnant within 6 months of trying. Within the first year, 80 to 90 percent of couples should have conceived. However, the exact length of time to conception varies greatly with age.

How common are fertility problems experienced?

Around 1 in 7 couples suffer from fertility problems.

If a woman managed to conceive previously but has problems conceiving again, she is said to have 'secondary infertility'. This may affect 1 in 10 couples. In such cases, it is possible that she has developed a new underlying health problem.

What causes infertility?

One-third of causes can be attributed to problems in the woman, another third of causes are due to problems in the man. The remaining third may be issues relating to both the woman and the man. Sometimes, no obvious cause can be found.

Female infertility factors

These can broadly be divided into 1) ovulation disorders e.g., hormonal disorders such as polycystic ovarian syndrome; 2) endometriosis where the lining of the uterus occurs outside its normal position e.g., at the back of the uterus and around the ovaries; 3) problems with the uterus e.g., fibroids and polyps; and 4) tubal disease which prevent the sperm from meeting and fertilising the egg.

Male infertility factors

In men, common causes include poor sperm count and/or poor sperm quality. This in turn could be due to an unhealthy lifestyle, smoking, or a previous infection. Certain cancers can also affect fertility and treatment of cancer with chemotherapy and radiation can impair fertility.

Who is at risk of infertility?

The following are risk factors for infertility:

Advanced age (over 35yrs): Age is a major factor especially in women. Other factors include their general state of health, diet and lifestyle.

Menstrual problems: Women who have irregular or painful periods may be at risk of fertility problems. If a woman has a history of irregular periods, this could indicate an ovulation problem where the egg is not released from the ovary regularly every month and will reduce her chances of conception. If she has painful periods, this may indicate the presence of a gynaecological problem such as endometriosis, ovarian cysts or fibroids which may prevent the implantation of a healthy embryo in the uterus.

Past medical or surgical history: A past history of infection resulting in pelvic inflammatory disease (PID), or previous surgery, may cause tubal disease which would prevent the egg and the sperm from meeting.

Poor diet and lifestyle choices: Smoking, alcohol use, being overweight or underweight can all affect fertility.

How does a woman's age influence her fertility? What are some statistics on conception rates for women in their 20s versus women in their 30s and 40s?

Age is an important contributing factor to infertility. Older women tend to have reduced fertility and are more likely to require fertility treatment for conception.

In women, fertility declines steadily with age. Women are born with a fixed number of eggs. With increasing age, there is a fall in the number of eggs left in the ovaries.

The likelihood of conceiving falls from 20 percent a month in a fertile 30-year-old woman to less than 5 percent at age 40. Even the success rate of artificial reproductive treatment is not spared and pregnancy rates fall with increasing age.[1]

Age is also an important contributing factor to male infertility. Although the evidence is less strong compared to women, men may also become less fertile as they get older. In men, the quantity and quality of sperm may deteriorate with time, making it difficult for them to reach and fertilise an egg. This can occur as a result of poor diet or lifestyle habits as well as chronic illnesses such as diabetes and raised blood pressure.

The term 'ovarian reserve' refers to a woman's current supply of eggs, and is closely associated with reproductive potential. In general, the younger the woman, the greater the number of eggs she has in her reserve, hence the better the chance for conception. Conversely, a low ovarian reserve greatly diminishes a patient's chances for conception.

Are we able to measure our 'ovarian reserve'?

Measuring the ovarian reserve is possible and useful in the evaluation for infertility patients.

The tests currently available for assessing ovarian reserve include ultrasound scans of the ovaries and blood tests for female hormones such as the Anti-Müllerian Hormone (AMH), a hormone produced by the eggs in the ovaries. As the number of eggs falls, there is a concurrent decrease in the AMH levels. AMH can therefore be measured to give an indication of the ovarian reserve.

It has been recommended that ovarian reserve testing be performed for women older than 35 years, those who have not conceived after 6 months of trying, and for those at higher risk of diminished ovarian reserve.

When results indicate a poor reserve, a patient may be counselled that her window of opportunity to conceive may be shorter than expected and she should attempt to conceive sooner rather than later, or consider fertility treatment earlier.

How does a woman's age affect her pregnancy risks?

Pregnancy in women of advanced age over 35 years has been associated with an increased risk of complications. For the mother, complications include gestational diabetes, hypertension and caesarean section. Older women are also more likely to suffer a miscarriage.

Do miscarriages contribute significantly to the low birth rate in Singapore?

15 to 20 percent of pregnancies end in a miscarriage. It is probably being reported more as couples these days plan actively and know very early on that they are pregnant. But there may also be an increase in the number of miscarriages now because more women are delaying childbearing to an older age and we know that the risk of miscarriages increases with age.

With increasing age, our general health also tends to decline. Existing conditions may worsen or new illnesses may develop, which can also have an impact on fertility. In addition, there is also a decline in quality of eggs and an increased risk of genetic abnormalities. This in turn results in an increased risk of miscarriage. The risk of a miscarriage is around 15 percent for a woman in her early 30s. This increases to around 25 percent for women 35–39 years, and climbs further to over 40 percent for women over 40 years.

What are some of the causes of miscarriages?

Miscarriages are most commonly due to genetic defects in the developing embryo. Genetic defects may occur as a result of fertilisation of unhealthy eggs or sperm. Miscarriages may also occur due to problems such as uterine anomalies and cervical incompetence. Couples should undergo investigations if they have had recurrent miscarriages i.e., more than 2 or 3 consecutive miscarriages.

Smoking, excess weight and physical inactivity have all been linked to difficulties in conception. How do these lifestyle factors influence fertility?

In women, smoking is harmful to the ovaries, accelerates egg loss, and may advance the age of menopause by several years. Studies indicate that smoking can predispose a woman's eggs to genetic abnormalities and increases the risk of miscarriage and possibly ectopic pregnancy. Smoking is also associated with an increased risk of cervical cancer which can affect fertility indirectly. In men, smoking is associated with abnormalities in sperm production, quality and quantity. Smoking can also lead to impotence by causing damage to blood vessels, resulting in weak and ineffective erections.

Being either overweight or underweight are both not ideal for fertility. Being underweight can reduce fertility, by decreasing the chances of implantation of the embryo in the uterus. Being obese is well-documented to also impair fertility and may also lead to irregular menstrual cycles and irregular ovulation.

Under-exercising and being overweight can also be bad for ovulation. However, over-exercising, e.g. over 60 minutes every day, can actually prevent ovulation. This is seen in athletes who stop having regular menstruation. Ideally, try to engage in moderate aerobic exercise — 30 to 40 minutes several times a week.

When trying to get pregnant, how often should couples be trying? Is there anything else they should be aware of?

Ideally, the frequency of intercourse should be 2 to 3 times a week.

For couples trying to get pregnant naturally, the most effective time to have sex is during the 'fertile window'. This window period includes the 5 days leading up to, and the day of, ovulation, when your body releases an egg. Your egg will survive for about a day once released from the ovary. But sperm can survive for up to 5 days. Hence there is a 6-day window for sperm to meet an egg.

However, having regular sex every 2 to 3 days throughout the month is generally advisable as this improves the quality of sperm compared to prolonged periods of abstinence.

When should couples seek professional help?

After one year of trying, if they still have not conceived, further investigations are warranted.

However, couples should seek advice earlier if they have risk factors for fertility problems e.g., menstrual problems or past medical or surgical history which may impact fertility.

Couples should also seek advice earlier if they are in the older age group, especially if the woman is over age 35. Such couples should be referred to a fertility specialist after 6 months of trying to get pregnant.

In view of the impact of age, early diagnosis and treatment are crucial to the successful management of infertility.

How do doctors determine if couples have an infertility problem?

During the medical consultation, a thorough medical history will be taken from the couple. This will be followed with investigations. For the woman, these would usually include a pelvic ultrasound scan, hormone blood tests, and a tubal patency test to assess the fallopian tubes for blockages. For the man, a semen analysis will be required.

How can infertility be treated?

Infertility can be treated depending on the cause. Some examples are discussed below:

Hormonal problems

Hormonal problems can cause failure to ovulate. Hormonal disorders may be caused by polycystic ovary syndrome or any problem related to the 'Hypothalamic-Pituitary-Ovarian axis' — where hormones act in turn to stimulate the ovaries to release an egg every month. Symptoms of lack of ovulation include irregular cycles. Depending on the specific hormone disorder, there may be specific symptoms e.g., hyperthyroidism (too much thyroid hormone) can cause palpitations and weight loss; hyperprolactinaemia (too much prolactin hormone) can cause milk secretions from the breasts.

Treatment will depend on the exact underlying type of hormone problem which will need to be treated accordingly. Sometimes, treatment of the underlying problem will result in normalisation of the ovulation cycle.

For problems related to abnormal ovulation: fertility drugs or hormone injections may help to enable ovulation to occur in a more predictable manner. Ultrasound scans may also be performed in the clinic to help determine more precisely when ovulation will occur. Urine tests to measure the presence of a luteinizing hormone (LH) surge which occurs before ovulation, can also be useful to time ovulation. Advice can then be given as to when the best time for sexual intercourse would be, to maximise fertilisation chances.

Endometriosis

This is a condition where the lining of the uterus is deposited outside the uterine cavity, possibly around the ovaries, resulting in the development of ovarian cysts. Symptoms include severe menstrual pain and pain during intercourse. Endometriosis also decreases pregnancy success rates due to the inflammation around the uterus and ovaries.

Treatment involves laparoscopy and cystectomy with surgical removal of endometriotic lesions. Laparoscopy involves insertion of a fine telescope through the umbilicus and the use of long and slim instruments. The skin incisions are very small (around 5mm) and recovery is usually fast. After surgery, hormonal treatment is sometimes needed to suppress the recurrence of endometriosis before fertility treatment is started.

Uterus irregularities

Uterine irregularities may prevent the embryo from implanting well inside the uterus. Problems include the presence of a septum — which is a band of excess tissue which divides the uterus. Other problems include large fibroids or endometrial polyps.

Treatment will depend on the nature of the problem. For problems such as a uterine septum, submucous fibroids which distort the uterine cavity, or endometrial polyps, hysteroscopy may be performed to treat the problem. This involves insertion of a fine telescope through the vagina into the uterus. The uterine cavity can then be cleared to optimise conditions for implantation of the embryo.

Poorly functioning fallopian tubes

The fallopian tubes may be damaged and prevent the sperm and egg from meeting. Causes of tubal damage include a past history of pelvic infection or previous surgery which can cause inflammation and scarring of tubes. Sometimes, the fallopian tubes may not have been formed normally during development. A damaged tube may also lead to ectopic pregnancy where the embryo sticks inside the tube instead of implanting in the uterus.

Treatment will depend on severity of the tubal damage. Sometimes, surgery may help to unblock tubes. However, if a tube is badly damaged and swollen, it may need to be removed as it can cause a decrease in the pregnancy success rates with fertility treatment.

Sperm production/quality/motility

Sperm production/quality and mobility can be affected by the general health of the man. Medical illness and medication can affect the sperm. Unhealthy diets and lifestyles can also affect the sperm.

Treatment depends on severity of the sperm count and quality. A referral to a urologist may be recommended to assess for the presence of abnormalities which can be surgically treated e.g., varicocoeles. Sometimes, lifestyle and diet modification may be prescribed e.g., smoking cessation, and a trial of vitamin supplements and antioxidants may be helpful. Ultimately, assisted reproductive methods such as intra-uterine insemination (IUI) or in-vitro fertilisation (IVF) can help bypass male factor fertility.

What is IUI and who should consider it?

Intra-uterine insemination (IUI) is a more 'natural' form of fertility treatment. IUI may be considered if the fallopian tubes are both healthy with no blockages, and there are at least 1 million motile sperm on semen analysis.

What does IUI involve?

IUI involves the preparation of a semen sample and injection of the sample directly into the uterus using a fine catheter. The IUI process helps to 'wash' the sperm so that the more motile sperm is obtained for injection into the uterus. It also helps to bring the sperm closer to the egg, bypassing the vaginal and cervical mucus factors that may prevent the sperm from swimming into the uterus.

What is the success rate of IUI?

IUI success rates are around 15 percent per cycle, comparable to trying naturally if there are no fertility problems, but lower compared with IVF. It is often recommended that if suitable for IUI, a couple consider IUI first before progressing to IVF.

What is IVF and who should consider it?

In-vitro fertilisation (IVF) refers to the use of laboratory techniques to bring the egg and sperm together outside of the woman's body. IVF is well-established as the most effective mode of infertility treatment, particularly where the female fallopian tubes are blocked and/or the male sperm count is low. By overcoming the potential problems that prevent fertilisation of the egg with the sperm at the microscopic level, IVF helps to provide the highest pregnancy success rate for a couple.

Couples may be advised to consider IVF earlier if the woman's fallopian tubes are blocked, preventing natural conception, or if the sperm number and quality are very poor. They may also be advised to consider IVF if the woman is in the older age group and/or has a limited ovarian reserve and they wish to have a higher success rate than IUI. Depending on the fertility factors at play, couples may be advised to move directly to IVF.

What is the success rate of IVF?

The success rate for IVF is mostly female age-dependent. Generally, the pregnancy success rate for IVF is around 50 percent for the younger age group under 40 years, but falls once the woman reaches 40 years and above.[2]

IVF success rates can also be affected by the presence of other gynaecological factors such as endometriosis, ovarian cysts, uterine fibroids and polyps. Surgery may therefore still be recommended to increase the IVF treatment success.

What does IVF involve?

IVF treatment involves several different steps. Firstly, in order to increase the number of eggs produced by her ovaries, the woman has to undergo hormonal injections. For ovarian stimulation, different protocols for different women are available. Secondly, ultrasound scans and blood tests are needed to assess the growth and maturity of the eggs. Once the eggs are ready, they are retrieved with the help of a vaginal ultrasound while the woman is under anaesthesia. The eggs are then fertilised with the sperm in the laboratory to form embryos before they are transferred back into the woman's womb.

What are some complications of IVF treatment?

Complications are uncommon but there may be side effects with the use of various hormone treatments. With fertility drugs, some side effects include abdominal bloating, nausea, headaches and tiredness. There is also a risk of multiple pregnancy, such as twins, especially if more than one embryo is transferred back into the uterus.

With fertility hormone injections, problems include psychological stress and physical discomfort. Egg retrieval which is performed under anaesthesia entails some small risks of anaesthesia, bleeding and infection. With the rise in hormone levels in the body, there may be a risk of 'ovarian hyperstimulation syndrome' or OHSS. This condition can result in nausea, vomiting and dehydration, and may require hospitalisation. Hence, close monitoring, care and medical attention are important.

Is there hope for fertility in cancer patients?

Treatments for cancer — such as chemotherapy and radiotherapy — may damage fertility. In such cases, sperm and eggs can be frozen before treatment starts, in order to prolong fertility.

Recent advances in cancer therapy have resulted in an increased number of long-term cancer survivors. Quality of life is an important issue for cancer survivors and fertility after cancer treatment is often a concern. With the recent success and advances made in fertility preservation for cancer patients, international guidelines now recommend that these options should be discussed with the patient. If a young patient is diagnosed with cancer, it is important to let them know early about such possibilities. The strategies to preserve fertility in women with cancer include frozen storage of embryos, storage of oocytes for future in-vitro fertililisation, and storage of ovarian tissues.

Freezing of embryos

Freezing of embryos is the most established technique but requires ovarian stimulation, oocyte retrieval and in-vitro fertilisation, which takes about 2 to 5 weeks. This may not be practical for many cancer patients. It is also not an option for pre-pubertal girls and women who do not have a partner. However, if circumstances allow, freezing of embryos is the most reliable method for improving pregnancy success rates later.

Freezing of eggs

Freezing of mature eggs requires ovarian stimulation and will also delay cancer therapy. Without ovarian stimulation, a number of immature oocytes may be retrieved. These immature oocytes may undergo maturation in-vitro before freezing by vitrification. Vitrification refers to a method of 'rapid freezing' to prevent ice crystal formation in the eggs which tends to destroy the egg cells.

Freezing of ovarian tissue

In recent years, there have been an increasing number of reports of successful restoration of fertility after auto-transplantation of frozen and thawed ovarian tissue. For such cases, before cancer treatment is commenced, ovarian tissue is surgically removed and frozen. Following treatment of the cancer, if the patient is diagnosed to have premature menopause and is keen to get pregnant, the frozen ovarian tissue is thawed and transplanted back into the patient.

What are some lifestyle habits we can adopt to improve fertility?

Regarding lifestyle habits:

- Couples who smoke should stop smoking — smoking impairs sperm quality and female smokers are more likely to experience earlier menopause before age 50 due to the effect of tobacco toxins on the reproductive system.
- Limit alcohol intake — in women, there is no 'safe' level of alcohol use during conception or pregnancy. Heavy drinking of more than 7 drinks a week and binge drinking of more than 3 drinks in a sitting can harm fertility through impact on liver function and hormone function. For men, heavy alcohol use can decrease sperm count and motility.
- Limit coffee intake to 1–2 cups a day — high levels of caffeine (more than 400mg a day) may be associated with decreased fertility and increased risks of miscarriage.
- Try to start planning for a family as early as possible.
- Maintain a normal weight, exercise and eat a diet rich in fruits, vegetables and antioxidants.

  For women:

- Take folic acid to prevent certain birth defects like spina bifida.
- It may be useful to visit a doctor for a 'preconception' check to review what can be done to optimise the chances of a successful pregnancy.

  For men:

- Wear loose-fitting undergarments.
- Avoid extremely hot temperatures, such as hot tubs or saunas. High temperatures can affect sperm production and motility.

Further Reading

Age and Fertility: A Guide for Patients. Reproductive Facts by the American Society for Reproductive Medicine; 2012. Available at https://docs.google. com/viewer?url=https%3A%2F%2Fwww.reproductivefacts. org%2Fglobalassets%2Frf%2Fnews-and-publications%2Fbookletsfact-sheets%2Fenglish-fact-sheets-and-info-booklets%2FAge_and_Fertility.pdf

Fertility Problems: Assessment and Treatment. Clinical Guideline CG156. National Institute for Health and Care Excellence; 2017 Sep 6. Available at https://www.nice.org.uk/guidance/CG156.

CHALLENGES OF A WORKING MOTHER

Take Home Points

1. A working mother refers to a woman who juggles both the demands of home and the workplace.
2. It is very common for a working mother to feel a strong sense of guilt, either about not spending enough time with her child(ren), or not doing more at work.
3. A working mother oftentimes makes sacrifices so as to meet all the demands of her, resulting in deficits in her quality of life.
4. Self-care and a strong support system is key to surviving life as a working mother.
5. It is important to remember what works for the working mother and her family, and to avoid comparison with other mothers and/or working adults.

Dr Kim Lian Rolles-Abraham is a Senior Clinical Psychologist and Head of Therapy Services, specializing in Eating Disorders and General Psychology, and is currently practising at Better Life Psychological Medicine Clinic.

As I sat down and contemplated the task of writing this chapter, it dawned on me that this very process was reflective in so many ways of one of the struggles of a working mother. Juggling a multitude of work-related tasks and childcare duties, I was spectacularly late in delivering my piece on this topic.

What is a working mother?

A working mother is a woman who identifies with both the role of worker and mother. She plays a role in the care of her children (and oftentimes the affairs of the home) and works for an income in addition to that. It is pertinent to understand that both of these roles are extremely demanding, and that it is no mean feat trying to do right by both without neglecting some aspect of either of them.

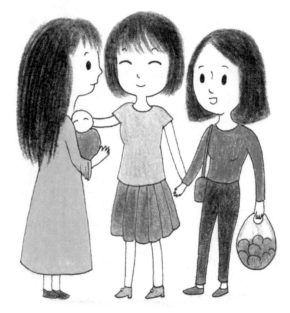

Societal Norms and Pressures

In spite of the huge shift toward dual income-earning households, women still bear the brunt of disproportionate childcare and household duties as mothers are expected to pour their energies into caring for their children The role of father, however, is often still seen as being a breadwinner, although this is changing in some societies.

However, this universally recognised intensive mothering concept seems to be incompatible with the normative expectations associated with the ideal worker. Good workers are expected to be unwaveringly committed to their employer/company at the expense of any other non-work obligation. In the same way, the ideal mother is not supposed to divide her time, energy and attention between her children and paid work. As such, the merging of the roles of being a mother and worker with mutually exclusive role expectations can create huge conflicts for working mothers.

The Decision to Become a Working Mother

One does not just *become* a working mother. The challenges inherent in the role of a working mother start at the very beginning; the decision-making process that ultimately results in the decision to care for a child and work for income at the same time.

When a woman becomes a working mother, she is either pushed or pulled into the decision. For some individuals, it is a necessity — there is no option, because the mother (and the family, as a unit) requires additional income to subsist on. For others, it is a choice (which in some cases reflects a necessity) — some women enjoy their work and relish in their role as a worker, and have seen how continuing to engage in meaningful work has knock-on benefits for their role as parent. Regardless of whether a mother engages in work because she needs to or wants to, this does not come without its associated challenges.

Work

We have seen a steady rise in the number of women who have joined the workforce in the last few decades. According to figures from the Singapore Department of Statistics,[1] female labour force participation in Singapore was 58.1 percent in 2013, from 28.2 percent in 1970. Despite it being more commonplace to have women at the workplace, working mothers continue to face challenges in their jobs that are unique to them as employees.

The challenges they face include how they feel at work themselves, how they are made to feel at work by others, and the support, or lack thereof that they receive at the workplace.

While working at a pace that allows for both the benefits of money and time with children, many mothers experience disappointment in losing out on opportunities in career advancement. This can occur due to several factors, including time lost during maternity leave, sometimes a preference towards giving a work role to someone who would be less inclined to have their time divided between work and family. To bridge the cognitive dissonance that some mothers experience, they may choose to deny their career aspirations and detach emotionally from anything work-related while channelling their efforts into the care of their children.

Career Progression Opportunities

Some working mothers find the pathway for career progression more arduous than their male counterparts. There is the perception that the working mother would have greater work-family conflicts and hence also doubts about whether they would be able to juggle all their home responsibilities, as well as give their all at the workplace. The higher the work-family conflicts, women managers report, the greater the stress, depression and irritation.[2] Hence, it would be easier for an employer to pass a working mother up for a promotion as there would be doubts about long-term commitments and willingness to go the extra mile to help the organization succeed, given the other priorities constantly competing for the attention of the working mother. There is a fear among some employers that the chances of the working mother needing to take urgent family care leave in the event that a family member falls sick is higher, compared to other employees. These family responsibilities such as household tasks, marriage and childcare have been shown to slow down/impede the achievements of women managers.[3]

Sense of Mastery

As the working mother has to juggle several roles at the same time, i.e., being a mother, wife and worker, this could obviously create a strain even as she tries to do the best she can. Despite equal career demands for both men and women, women managers rarely receive sufficient support and help from society and organisations.[4]

Working mothers however (like most other human beings) want to be recognised for the work they do — which consists of both the work at home (child-related work) as well as at the workplace (job-related work). It is usually difficult to get recognised if the work is not done 'well enough'. It is also usually difficult to do work 'well enough', when you have got split priorities; working mothers are often made to feel like a jack-of-all-trades, but the masters of none. As they tirelessly chase their tails picking up after their children and tying up loose ends at work, their sense of mastery and satisfaction with what they do can be quite diminished. Job fulfilment starts to wane when the working mother is aware that more could have been made out of a project, but compromises had to be made as her attention was divided. The lack of time may also hinder the working mother from getting the necessary support, training and mentoring that might aid her in honing her craft and upgrading her skills. Senior figures at work may also not want to invest the extra time and energy to provide additional support for the working mother compared to a regular employee and this in itself could emerge as a source of irritation.

As a young clinical psychologist, I felt my career slipping like sand through my fingers as I watched my peers skyrocket ahead of me — taking on greater caseloads and availing themselves to more 'extracurricular activities' that resulted in an overall boost in their professional eligibility. I was branded as not having the bandwidth, and told countless times that the world would be my oyster, "when you stop getting pregnant" and "when your children get older". I was shown, essentially, that being a mother was a limiting factor. As someone who had desired having children very much, I balked at my unforeseen thoughts and feelings of resentment towards my children in light of my perceived dwindling career.

I recall distinctly, a moment when I was holding my 14-month-old in my arms while using my right foot to rock the rocking chair of my 3-month-old. I asked myself, "Is this what I studied a doctorate to do?" As one-dimensional as that thought was, it was very real and very intense. Of course, motherhood comes with its joys, but every now and then, such thoughts can creep in and threaten to shake my equanimity.

Logistical Concerns Pertaining to Motherhood

The reality of working mothers is that the responsibilities of motherhood cannot always be left at home. One example would be breastfeeding and the pumping of breast milk that needs to be maintained throughout the day. Not all workplaces are equipped with a room where the mother can go to pump breast milk at the right time. Not all employers would be sympathetic to a mother having to pause her work mid-task, to go and pump milk. These are just some of the minefields that a working mother has to navigate when they are trying to maintain the role of both being a new mother and an employee.

The mother may also be the person coordinating the care of the child while being away from home, in terms of organising the logistics of child care, be it with a helper, grandparent or another relative. Some mothers may feel the need to be cautious and have CCTV cameras installed at home to monitor their helpers, especially if the helper is new or has had previous work ethic concerns. This would be an additional 'home' situation that would need to be brought to work to some extent, hence possibly dividing the mother's attention at the workplace.

Feelings of Guilt

Guilt, shame and the perennial feeling of being 'not good enough' is something many working mothers struggle with as they try to divide their time and energy appropriately between their various undertakings. The sacrifices mothers make are immeasurable — they give up their bodies, time, sleep, finances, social lives, careers and preferences (amongst other things) for their children. In spite of everything they trade in and even when it seems like there is nothing else they could have done better or differently, the question often remains: *"Am I good enough?".*

Where does guilt and shame come from? The same place the feeling of not being good enough comes from — comparison. According to social comparison theory,[5] we determine our personal and social worth on the basis of how we measure up to others. Upward social comparison (using those deemed 'better' than us as a benchmark) makes us feel like failures — although in some cases, it can be healthy motivation; downward social comparison (using those deemed 'worse off' than us as a benchmark) is our way of making ourselves feel better. As human beings, the proclivity to evaluate ourselves against a social benchmark is not only instinctual but also inculcated — from a young age, we are not only asked by our parents how we did in a test, but how the rest of our class did as well. We take part in competitions that reveal our standing in comparison to other participants. We are graded on a bell curve. The list goes on. If ensuring one's own success and taking care of oneself already involves so many social pressures, taking charge of another life form doubles or even triples it. In the land of Motherhood, social comparison takes on a life of its own.

Such feelings start to form even well before the child is brought into this world. Upon knowledge of successful conception, mothers are catapulted into the complex world of motherhood, and have to start making potentially guilt-inducing decisions — Do I keep the baby? Is my lifestyle causing harm to the foetus and do I need to make significant changes? Do I want to try for a natural birth or a c-section? Do I breastfeed, pump or use infant formula? Should I sleep train? Do I co-sleep? What brand of products should I purchase for my baby? Should I go organic? Sugar-free? No screen time? The questions are relentless, and it doesn't help when everyone other than the mother wants in on the decision-making process.

Even well-intentioned suggestions and comments from loved ones or formal recommendations from doctors can result in feelings of guilt, inadequacy and confusion. A burnt-out working mother may receive advice from her mental health professional to get more sleep for self-care, while her paediatrician tells her to pump every two hours to keep up milk supply, at the same time making sure that the baby is adequately and appropriately stimulated (without caving in to screen time).

Many first-time mothers today possess the amazing double-edged sword (that is both gift and curse) of too much knowledge. We use smart, fancy apps to track our child's development and worry endlessly when something seems slightly off or different from our friends' same age babies. We are inundated with social media posts and articles that teach us how to be a *better* parent. We spend our time and energy on any enrichment class or activity purported to boost our child's ability and give him an edge in life. There is pressure (be it external or internal) to keep up with other mothers who seem to be doing things right.

As I sit and write this, my children are watching 'PJ Masks' on Netflix — the only way I can possibly ensure that my one, two and three-year-olds (yes, you read that right) are safely preoccupied as I work — while I make note from social media that my friends' children are engaged in various homeschooling activities such as painting a home-made cardboard cut-out of the human body and practising writing their ABCs. I would be lying if I said I didn't feel even the tiniest bit of guilt.

In a case of being "damned if you do, damned if you don't", working mothers not only experience guilt when they feel like they are not doing enough with and for their children, but also when they feel like they are not doing enough at work. The problem with having competing needs is feeling like you're never meeting any of them well enough; I contradict myself on an almost-daily basis, swinging from deeply believing that I need to take that extra work call to feeling assured that bringing my children to the playground is the best decision. While on the work call, a part of me wonders if I could have forgone it to spend the last thirty minutes before sundown with my children and conversely, when I am at the playground, thoughts about whether I could have responded to another five emails creep into my mind.

Attachment Formation, Subjective and Objective Closeness to Her Child(ren)

Something else that could potentially spark guilt for a working mother is how close she feels she is to her child.

Bowlby[6] was among the first to study the importance of early relationships on later social and emotional development for children. He described how attachment behaviours stem from the biological drive to elicit responses from a caregiver, which would promote the infant-caregiver proximity. One of the primary dimensions of the development of attachment in humans is the concept of attachment formation.[7] This describes the extent to which a child differentiates familiar adults in his/her life from each other, showing a preference for one caregiver over another.

If a mother works, some of the childcare responsibilities may be outsourced to others, which would reduce the time a mother can spend with her child to develop a strong connection. While this is the reality of the situation, societal norms and expectations dictate otherwise, and there is the unspoken expectation that mothers ought to spend the most time with their child. In the Asian context where grandparents and the extended family are often an integral part of the support and caregiving network, many children of working parents are raised partly by them. Alternatively, children of working parents spend much of their waking hours at a childcare centre or with hired domestic help at home.

Given that children are being cared for by adults other than their mothers while their mothers focus on work, it is understandable that the children start developing attachments to their other carers, sometimes seemingly at the expense of attachment to their mothers. This can then lead to internal struggles being faced by the mother — she has to battle the expectations of society and relatives, the desire to pursue fulfilment in her career and her own expectations and judgements of herself. There have been seasons during which I have worked longer hours, and as my baby saw me less, she naturally preferred other caregivers who spent more time with her. I distinctly recall how it felt each time I reached out to pick my baby up, only to have her violently recoil from me and turn in the direction of my domestic helper, indicating quite blatantly her preference of caregiver. Fortunately, as I have learned, some of these experiences are typically time-limited, reflecting a cross-section of intense demands all around.

Spousal/Sexual Relationship

For some men, the very fact that their wives work can cause strain in the relationship. Following the industrial revolution, there was a division of home and work into separate spheres which led to the concept of the male breadwinner which denoted the exclusive male responsibility to provide for the family. A "good provider" was historically described as a "man whose wife did not enter the labour force".[8] The man's responsibility to provide for the family was juxtaposed with the woman's responsibility to care for the home and family. Zelizer demonstrated how money earned by married women in the labour market was often deemed as supplementary income and treated as less important than their husbands' salaries.[9] The concept of defining the wife's income as supplementary diminishes the threat to the male breadwinner ideal as it does not challenge the man's position as the financial provider for the family. This however becomes harder to do in modern times, especially in families where the wife is earning about the same as, if not more than, the husband. This could potentially impact on the identity of the man as he perceives that he is losing his grip on the role of primary provider for the family, resulting in conflict and tension in their spousal relationship.

As the mother works and attends to the needs of the household, her stress and fatigue levels can also have an impact on how sexual she feels, and sometimes she may want and need sleep a lot more than physical intimacy with her partner. Additionally, some mothers, after bearing a child for 9 months in their wombs, and experiencing a whole host of physiological changes, as well as a child clinging to them for breastfeeding or comfort, just want some space between their bodies and other human beings. This new state of affairs may result in frustration for the woman who used to enjoy romance/sex and overall dissatisfaction in the couple's relationship. She may also experience guilt for not meeting her husband's needs, especially as she watches him labour out of the home and help out in the home as well.

Self-care — Nutrition, Sleep, Exercise, Social Life

Nutrition

A working mother often feels rushed, working against the clock to strike a balance between her work and her family on a day-to-day basis. As such, she may very well end up compromising on what is necessary to fuel her pace of life. Some are nutritionally deficient, as they skip meals or make do with snacks on the go or fast food. A survey by the Working Mother Research Institute revealed that 44 percent of working mothers do not get time to sit down and have their meals, with statistics showing that the average working mother gets about 3 minutes and 15 seconds to eat breakfast and that she mostly eats it standing up.

Sleep

It is well documented that women experience significant sleep deprivation once they become mothers.

The negative impact that being a mother has on sleep quality probably begins even before the baby is born — when one's bladder is compressed and the discomfort of the physical changes due to the pregnancy are unbearable — and this impact lasts well past kindergarten. However, children waking throughout the night is not the only reason why mothers get so little sleep. Many working mothers, having devoted the day time to their work and their households, just want some time alone to decompress. This is often during the quiet of the night, when everyone else is sound asleep.

Ironically, sleep deprivation may result in a drop in performance at work, creating more stress, more things to do and worry about, which circle back to poor sleep again. It does not help that as a society, people tend to look down on sleep; rather than associating it with necessity, it gets tagged to indulgence. Some sleep-deprived mothers take pride in sleeping too little (for it must mean that they are getting heaps done in their wakeful state), and trade battle stories of sleepless nights with other weary mothers at the playground. This reinforces that sleepless mothering should be put on a pedestal and because 'she's doing it, so I too, can and must'. The social comparisons persist, even in a state of sleeplessness.

Exercise

Despite expressing the desire to exercise more, women with children display lower rates of physical activity compared to women without children, and working mothers are especially at risk of low levels of physical activity. Constraints around scheduling, guilt, poor social support, work demands and family commitments have been cited as prime obstacles to exercise in working mothers. In essence, working mothers often respond to the topic of exercise with "no time", or "too tired".

Exercise is a form of self-care as the benefits working mothers can experience from it are multi-fold. Not only is physical activity associated with a decreased risk for physical health issues, it also helps many women cope with the challenges of motherhood, restoring focus to themselves and giving them a respite from the demands of work and/or the family.

Social life

Motherhood can be terribly isolating and with the additional responsibility of work, it may mean that one has a lot less time for a social life. A working mother who juggles family and work may find that she has little or no time to develop or maintain an active social life. As her schedule revolves around her children's activities and her work-related tasks, it can be challenging to find a common time with her friends to meet. Certain times of the day are a no-go, as she either has to work or put her children to bed. What used to be dinner and drinks with friends is now replaced with bath and bedtime routines with sleep-resistant children. As such, she may lose some friendships, especially those wherein both parties are at different life stages.

Sometimes, her social life may be whittled down to the mothers of her children's playmates. While this definitely makes for much needed companionship, deep connections are not always easy to forge; conversations understandably revolve around the children they are either trying to soothe, clean up or chase after. Hence, playdates without real adult connection can leave a working mother feeling even more isolated, exhausted and resentful.

Mental health struggles

Finally, one of the results of feeling battle-weary from some or all of the abovementioned challenges is pregnancy-related mood and anxiety disorders. Postpartum depression can make mothers feel like no matter what decisions they make; they are doing it all wrong. Postpartum anxiety robs mothers of perspective, making it difficult to make good choices. Pre-existing mental health problems such as abandonment and childhood trauma may make it especially difficult for mothers to self-regulate and make sense of the uncomfortable emotions that may arise as a part of parenting.

Coping with these Challenges

Mindset shift

A shift away from viewing mother and worker as mutually exclusive, competing roles can be very helpful, i.e., understanding that both roles can co-exist in a meaningful way and that one can in fact benefit the other. Although the demands of both roles seem distinct and rather opposing, they can in fact enrich and inform each other. For example, by taking the perspective that the resources gained in one role can be reinvested in the other, and that experiences gained in one can enhance the experience of and performance in the other.

Some work-related experiences can foster positive parenting styles and beliefs that benefit the child's growth. Similarly, experiences of mothering can add to working women's professional lives — for example, research has shown that experience with childcare can enhance female managers' ability to lead and to demonstrate patience.[10] Therefore, by recognising the potential value in engaging in two seemingly conflicting roles, women can feel more empowered to take on the two concurrently.

Something's got to give — recognising that one cannot do everything perfectly

With competing demands, working mothers often find themselves spread thin; they don't have enough bandwidth to do everything, let alone to do everything well. Well, if being a working mother means that you're too tired and pressed for time to go through the process of a birthday-cake-making activity with your child, then in the grand scheme of things, settling for a store-bought cake is not going to make the child much worse off. Sometimes, dropping the ball in one arena is necessary to be able to pick up the other balls that are hurtling your way, and it is always ok to say, "I would have liked to, but I simply could not".

In the same vein, remembering that no parent is perfect is so important. That working mother whose Instagram account is choc-a-bloc with vivid accounts and photographs of her perfectly balanced worker and mother roles is likely also losing her cool behind the scenes; what we see is not always what we get.

Relinquishing control and asking for help

The African proverb "It takes a village to raise a child" holds especially true for working mothers who cannot spend a hundred percent of their time and energies on their children. Hence, identifying their village and harnessing its resources is a key part of the survival process. Once the village is identified, communicating clearly what one needs help with rather than assuming others 'should know' is important.

Additionally, relinquishing control can often mean receiving help when offered, not fretting about the small things around the house, and accepting that the help offered may not necessarily be a hundred percent in line with your own ideologies. When a working mother relies on the support of other caregivers, there will be times where conflicts can arise due to clashing views about how the care of the child should be carried out. It is important for the working mother to decide which battles are worth fighting and which 'negotiables' she can let go of. Asking for help in some cases may mean seeking out professional help, where necessary.

Figuring out what works for you and your family unit

Every family unit is different; we have different demands, beliefs, values, and resources. Not everything that is recommended to a mother will work for her, and neither is everything seemingly beneficial on social media necessary to incorporate. Speaking to your partner and/or other involved family members is key in coming to a common understanding on what is preferred, in spite of what is prescribed by society at large.

Drawing boundaries, saying no

Contrary to popular belief, 'no' can in fact be a loving word because the effects in the long run may beneficially outweigh saying 'yes' in that moment. In the heat of the moment, a guilt-ridden working mother is often hard-pressed to say 'yes'. It is ok to have insufficient bandwidth for everything that comes your way, and it is ok to turn others down, regardless of what they may think. Citing the commonly used analogy of putting one's own oxygen mask on first, a mother needs to put herself first to put her family first. It may sound like a simple concept for a mother to first take care of herself, but it has profound impact on how she is able to engage with her child and take care of him/her.

This may mean turning down a play date to attend to an urgent work task or saying no to a non-compulsory work event to spend more time with her child; a mother needs to be clear about what makes sense for her at the time of decision making. Sometimes, neither decision is a better one, but because a decision needs to be made anyway, a mother has to be resolute about it.

It is easy for mothers to forget this because once the baby arrives, friends and family shower the baby with gifts, cuddles and attention, reinforcing to the mother that the focus has now shifted from her to the baby; socialisation around welcoming the baby is symbolic of the notion that mothers need to think about and make decisions around the baby, even when it may cause them sadness or distress. Apart from self-care, the drawing of boundaries is, ironically, the factor that may save relationships, rather than saying yes under pressure and as a result allowing the relationship to fray due to built-up resentment over time.

Creative time management

Working mothers, being extremely pressed for time, have honed their ability to be creative. Some of us have figured out a way to get things done while getting other things done — taking a toddler out for a stroll can constitute exercise and childminding; bringing your child for a lunch date can count as connecting meaningfully with him/her while getting in good nutrition for yourself. Personally, I have learned to connect with friends or clear emails on my phone while in a taxi to or from work. I have also begun to take a child with me if I need to run errands.

Avoiding judgement and comparison

We judge ourselves and fear judgement because we judge others, projecting onto others the fears and the inadequacies which we experience within ourselves.

Being a mother (who also works) has been a humbling experience in that it has taught me not to judge other mothers. Every mother has her own set of struggles, and every child has different needs. We see photographs on social media or fleeting snapshots of mother-child interactions that do not paint the full picture. Full-time working mothers, part-time working mothers, stay-home mothers, single mothers, stepmothers and adoptive mothers each face very different challenges, all while trying to do what is best for their children and their families.

References

1. Singapore Department of Statistics. Annual Labour Force Participation Rate 2013. Retrieved from: http://www.singstat.gov.sg/statistics/browse_by_theme/economy/time_series/labour.xl
2. Greenglass ER, Burke RJ. Work and family precursors of burnout in teachers: Sex differences. *Sex Roles* 1988; 18(3): 215–229.
3. Gutek BA, Repetti RL, Silver DL. Nonwork roles and stress at work. In *Causes, Coping and Consequences of Stress at Work* (Volume 2), eds. Cooper CL, Payne R, Chichester: John Wiley & Sons (1988: pp. 141–174).
4. Davidson MJ, Cooper CL. Executive women under pressure. *J Appl Psychol* 1986; 35(3): 301–325; Madhavi C, Vimala B. A study on work related stress and work family issues experienced by women software professionals in Chennai. *International Proceedings of Economic Development and Research* 2011; 12: 264–268.
5. Festinger L. A theory of social comparison processes. *Human Relations* 1954; 7(2): 117–140.
6. Bowlby J. *Attachment and Loss* (Volume 1). New York: Basic Books (1969).
7. Carlson EA, Hostinar CE, Mliner SB, Gunnar MR. The emergence of attachment following early social deprivation. *Development and Psychopathology* 2014; 26(2): 479–489.
8. Bernard J. The good-provider role: Its rise and fall. *The American Psychologist* 1981; 36(1): 1–12.
9. Zelizer VA. *The Social Meaning of Money*. Princeton, NJ: Princeton University Press (1997).
10. Ruderman MN, Ohlott PJ, Panzer K, King S. Benefits of multiple roles for managerial women. *Academy of Management Journal* 2002; 45(2): 369–386.

CHALLENGES OF A WORKING MOTHER

Take Home Points

1. There is no perfect time for childbearing.
2. Come to terms with your decision to pursue a career and motherhood, and celebrate every small achievement in both your career and motherhood journey.
3. Intentionally set aside time for self care and apply stress management strategies that work for you, to maintain physical, mental and emotional wellness.
4. Career progression may be delayed with necessary breaks (e.g,. hospitalisation leave during a complicated pregnancy, maternity leave, no pay leave to manage childcare arrangements) but the health of the mother and child should not be compromised.
5. Motherhood is a privilege, though it involves much sacrifice. Always remember to take care of yourself so that you can extend care to those around you; do not be shy to ask for help when needed.

Dr Rachel Ng Qiao Ming is an Associate Consultant in the department of Geriatric Medicine, and is currently practising at the Singapore General Hospital.

Family Planning — Am I Ready?

Pursuing medical education as a second degree at the Duke-NUS Graduate Medical school was an intentional decision when I knew a second medical school was in the pipeline, shortly after my 'A' level results were released. Being much younger then, single and without much family commitments, I was determined to pursue my career aspirations. It did not occur to me that motherhood would change my perspective of life. Therefore, at my medical school interview in 2008, when asked if I had thought about family planning and whether I would give up my practice after childbearing, I was rather confident in my answer that I would continue pursuing my career in medicine because being a geriatrician has been my childhood aspiration and I would not want to put years of medical school education and training to waste by giving up my practice. At that point, I had not considered the need for family planning in the future.

Shortly after getting married in my 3rd year of medical school, I gave much more thought to family planning — when will I be ready? There was much apprehension, and I was not sure if it was the right time for me to bear children, because I was preparing to enter my final year of medical school, which included going for major exit exams and subsequently entering into housemanship cum internal medicine residency training programme, which is another realm of uncertainty, filled with greater responsibilities as a practising physician and a junior resident.

Based on historical data, most female doctors avoid getting pregnant or having to care for children during their housemanship year, as they would be practising on a provisional license while being at the lowest of the hierarchical chain. During this period, there is so much to familiarise oneself with — the healthcare system and work culture, while learning to translate medical knowledge acquired during medical school into practice, acquiring practical clinical experience and learning to manage expectations of the patients under your care and their family members. With much prayer and after consulting senior physicians in the field who have families of their own and listening to their experience, I came to the realisation that there is actually no perfect time to start a family and raise children. Being a physician who is working in an institution, as my career progresses on, more responsibilities would be bestowed upon me. The ability to juggle work and family responsibilities would not get any easier. Furthermore, delaying childbirth to an age when morbidity is higher, fertility has decreased due to the physiological effects of aging, and having a higher risk of labour and delivery complications may not be ideal. With that in mind, my husband and I had greater peace to start growing our family when God blessed us with child. With much prayer, I conceived 4 months before my medical school's final exams, started housemanship when I entered my 3rd trimester of pregnancy, and delivered just shy of 3 months after commencing my junior residency programme.

Clinical Work and Residency Training During Pregnancy

As with various stages of motherhood, this journey of trying to protect the pregnancy in the midst of juggling clinical work and residency training, and with the aim to perform my duties well, was a constant struggle. There were many patients to review daily, both before and during consultant rounds, as well as post rounds to follow up with necessary changes. Our team's patients were scattered across all 4 blocks of the hospital at various floors. A lot of time was spent walking from one patient to another to review and optimise patient care and work hours were also long. Often times my basic needs of food, water, toileting and sleep were inadequately met. I was also at risk of contracting infectious diseases simply due to my environmental exposure, also known as occupational hazard. Moreover, knowing how close my estimated date of delivery (EDD) was to the end of my first 3 months posting, I was afraid a spontaneous early delivery would penalise me from completing my residency training posting, resulting in the need to repeat the entire posting upon returning from maternity leave. In addition, an earlier delivery would shorten the duration of my new employment, which would deny me the entitlement to paid maternity leave. With this calculated risk in mind, I persevered on through my posting without taking any leave in between, thinking I would buffer for an earlier delivery by taking my leave only towards the end of my posting. However, little did I expect to catch a bug that caused me to have severe diarrhoea at 35 weeks of my pregnancy. I was not only forced to take leave but also worry about the health of the foetus being compromised. After close monitoring of foetal movements in hospital for 2 days and supportive treatment, I was excited to return to work and continue to push on towards the goal of completing my posting before delivery. Unexpectedly, just a few days after being discharged from hospital, during my obgyn review, my baby's water bag level was noted to be very low, thus posing a threat to the life of my baby. I had to be readmitted for close monitoring of the foetal movements and was told to prepare for labour induction in the event that baby showed signs of distress. The struggle was real for me, I was totally unprepared — mentally, physically and emotionally, for the early arrival of my baby. Despite having contingency plans in advance, delivering at 36 or 37 weeks would mean that I would not be able to complete my 3-month posting within the maximum stipulated days of leave of absence and also not be entitled to paid maternity leave. These thoughts weighed against the health and safety of my baby even though to many, it may be obvious that priority should be the safeguarding of my foetus' health in the womb. Thankfully baby remained well throughout while under close foetal monitoring, and I had some time to sort of my thoughts before the repeat ultrasound scan of the water bag level for a final decision on labour induction. I was eventually at peace with the decision of labour induction because baby's health and safety should take precedence over my work commitments. Therefore, since the water bag level remained low on repeat scan, it was a sign from baby that he wanted to come out. Baby number 1 was delivered safely on September 21, 2013.

Coping with Miscarriages

Fast forward a year later, towards the end of my housemanship year, I was keen to try for another child. Unfortunately, the second and third pregnancies did not make it past the 12th week and I was extremely devastated each time I detected the loss of heartbeat in the foetuses. I felt that perhaps the hectic year of struggling to complete my housemanship while juggling motherhood responsibilities — nursing the child, maintaining the breastmilk supply and nurturing the child, despite persistent sleep deprivation — was simply damaging to my body. The loss of two consecutive pregnancies was an emotional roller coaster for me. On some days I would comfort myself that they were unhealthy pregnancies and that it was not God's will for me to have more babies midway through my residency training, given I was already struggling to complete the process. At other times I would simply cry at the thought of my losses and long for more children. I came to the realisation that although as a woman, successful childbearing was originally intended to be a primary role, in the midst of choosing to pursue other roles in life, I faced difficulty in fulfilling this primary role. This brought perspective to the priorities in my life and taught me how I should navigate life, moving forward, while fulfilling my multiple roles — as a wife, mother, a sibling, a child and a working professional, just to name a few.

Post-maternity Leave

After returning to work, I experienced constant struggle to manage post-maternity leave separation anxiety, maintain breastmilk supply at work, pick up the work and training where I had left off and recalibrate myself back to the work environment.

Having to juggle at least 3 separate roles as a new mother, a physician and a resident in training required seamless multi-tasking skills — the most efficient way around things. But certainly it also tired me out physically, mentally and emotionally. The expectations of others — my child, my spouse, my patients, my colleagues and seniors at work, on me, compounded the situation further.

A Physician and a Mother

The flip side to all the challenges I faced in being a physician and a mother is that my life has become even more exciting than it would have been, with the privilege of journeying through motherhood as a woman. Life is more exciting because it is hardly the same old routine that you will be going through at various stages of your child's development. Many times I have laughed so hard after being tickled by the little things my children say or do. Likewise, I have also cried buckets of tears during times I neglected them because of work commitments and they expressed their sadness from my absence. Motherhood is tough, especially with competing attention from other responsibilities, especially work commitments for working mothers, but I still do consider this added role an honour and privilege! In addition, the children have taught me so much about how I can be a better person. Though they have stretched my patience many times when they misbehaved, especially when I was extremely exhausted after work, I do feel challenged to be a better mother when I am with the children — to exhibit more love, patience, gentleness and grace. Personally, I have noted much similarity between the role of a physician and that of a mother, despite their obvious differences, one of being a caregiver. Being a caregiver to my patients and my children, it is important for me to take care of myself before extending myself as a caregiver to those under my care. Therefore, my advice to all the mothers pursuing professional careers is to take good care of yourself and be recharged so that you can carry out your multiple roles with greater tenacity, energy and fulfilment!

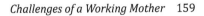
Further Reading

Finch SJ. Pregnancy during residency: A literature review. *Academic Medicine* 2003; 78 (4): 418–428.

Hoffman R, Mullan J, Nguyen M, Bonney AD. Motherhood and medicine: Systematic review of the experiences of mothers who are doctors. *MJA* 2020; 213(7): 329–333.

Serrano KD. On being a resident and a Mom. *Annals of Emergency Med* 2010; 55(5): 481–482.

MIDDLE-AGED WOMEN

SCREENING FOR CHRONIC CONDITIONS AND CANCER

Take Home Points

1. Get screened early and regularly even if you feel perfectly fine. Many diseases have no symptoms till late stages.
2. Get screened regularly even if you have no family history of any disease. Many diseases can be caused by environmental and lifestyle choices.
3. Heart disease in women is 6 times more common than breast cancer; hence do take care of your heart.
4. Most diseases result from a combination of genetic and lifestyle/ environmental factors. Though we cannot change our genetic disposition to diseases, we can change our lifestyles so as to be on a better path to good health.
5. Exercise at least 30 minutes daily. Eat a balanced diet. And most importantly, stay positive.

Dr Crystal Ng is a Family Physician, specializing in Health Screening, Occupational Health and Dermatology, and is currently practising at Fullerton Health at the Ocean Financial Centre.

Kids, spouse, parents, work, pets... Women have endless concerns from the many areas of our lives; very often, prioritising them before our own needs. Yet, there is one and only one of you in this world.

Taking good care of our physical, emotional and mental health is most important before we can take good care of our loved ones.

In this chapter, we will explore the most common conditions affecting women and how we can detect these conditions effectively.

Heart Disease

What is heart disease?

Heart disease includes a range of conditions affecting the heart, such as coronary artery disease, abnormal heart rhythms, heart valves and even infection of the heart.

Heart disease killed 6 times as many women as breast cancer in 2019.

The symptoms vary with the type of heart disease. Coronary heart disease is the most common type of heart disease. This is usually caused by a build-up of cholesterol plaque deposit in the arteries. A heart attack occurs when the blood supply to the heart muscles is completely blocked.

What are the signs and symptoms of a heart attack?

The symptoms may be very different for men and women. Men tend to have chest pain while women might not have any chest pain. Instead, they are more likely to have breathlessness, extreme fatigue, back pain, jaw pain or nausea. Up to one-quarter of all heart attacks are silent.

Am I at risk of getting it?

Hypertension, high blood cholesterol, diabetes, smoking, a lack of exercise, being overweight, stress, age, having a family history of heart disease and being of Indian ethnicity puts one at risk of contracting coronary heart disease.

Risk of heart disease also increases with menopause as the protective female hormone, oestrogen is reduced.

How do I detect it?

A resting electrocardiogram can detect heart muscle damage and abnormal rhythm; however, it might not show any blockages in the arteries.

An exercise stress treadmill test detects up to 70 percent of coronary heart disease while a CT (computed tomography) coronary angiogram looks at the arteries that supply blood to the heart. Discuss with your doctor on your risk factors and symptoms in order to decide on the best course of action.

What can I do to reduce my risk?

To reduce the risk, let's look at how we can reduce the risk factors mentioned above. Since we cannot change the non-modifiable risk factor such as family history and genetic predisposition to heart disease, we should actively look at the risk factors that we can change.

Better control of hypertension, diabetes, and high blood cholesterol is critical to reduce the risk of heart disease. Stop smoking and consuming alcohol. Engage in moderate intensity exercise for at least 150 minutes per week.

Consume plenty of vegetables, fruits, nuts, whole grains, lean animal protein and fish. Reduce intake of trans fats, red meat, refined carbohydrates and sweetened beverages.

Hyperlipidaemia

What is hyperlipidaemia?

Hyperlipidaemia means having high level of lipids (including cholesterol and triglycerides) in the blood. We need lipids for normal body functions. However, too much of it can cause coronary heart disease and stroke.

What are the signs and symptoms of hyperlipidaemia?

There are usually no signs or symptoms associated with hyperlipidaemia. However, over time, it might cause lipid plaque formation in the blood vessel walls leading to heart attack and stroke.

Am I at risk of getting it?

Our liver makes about 80 percent of the cholesterol in our bodies and the remainder comes from our diet — poultry, seafood, egg yolk, dairy products, and palm oil commonly found in baked products and ice-cream. Seafood such as crabs, lobsters, squids and prawns are also known to contain higher cholesterol.

Everyone aged 40 years and above should get screened for hyperlipidaemia. If you have first degree relatives diagnosed with familial hyperlipidaemia, screening can be carried out from age 2 years onwards. This encourages good eating practices from a young age.

If you have been diagnosed with coronary heart disease, stroke, diabetes/pre-diabetes, you should get screened for hyperlipidaemia.

How do I detect it?

A screening blood test for fasting/non-fasting lipids should be done every 3 years to check if you are within a normal range. Those at risk of coronary artery disease should do the blood test annually.

What can I do to reduce my risk?

Reduce dietary saturated fats found in red meat and full fat dairy products. Eliminate trans fats from your diet. Trans fats are typically found in baked products, fried fast food, margarine, hydrogenated vegetable oils, microwaveable popcorn and coffee creamers.

Increase your intake of vegetables, fruits, whole grains, fish, poultry, nuts and fibre.

Maintain a healthy weight. Engage in aerobic exercise for at least 4–5 times per week, each time lasting 30–45 minutes.

Quit smoking.

Hypertension

What is hypertension?

Hypertension is more commonly known as high blood pressure. Blood pressure is the pressure of blood pushing against the walls of the arteries. It is measured using two numbers. The first number is known as the systolic blood pressure. It measures the pressure when your heart contracts. The second number is known as the diastolic blood pressure. It measures the pressure when your heart relaxes.

In the United States, a normal blood pressure level is defined as less than 120/80 mmHg. In Singapore, we take the normal blood pressure to be below 130/85 mmHg.

High blood pressure occurs when your blood pressure is consistently higher than normal.

What are the signs and symptoms of hypertension?

Hypertension is also known as a silent killer as there are usually no warning signs or symptoms. The only way to diagnose it is to measure your blood pressure regularly.

Many people only come to know they have hypertension after a heart attack or stroke.

Am I at risk of getting it?

You are at risk if you have the following risk factors:

- Family history of hypertension
- Chronic kidney disease
- Obstructive sleep apnoea
- Stress
- Obesity
- Age
- Cigarette smoking
- Lack of exercise
- High salt diet
- Excessive alcohol consumption
- Stress
- Adrenal/thyroid gland disorders.

How do I detect it?

You can measure your blood pressure at home or visit a doctor. Do not smoke or drink caffeinated beverages 30 minutes before measuring your blood pressure. Empty your bladder. Sit still for 5 minutes before measuring. Ensure you sit upright with feet on the floor and legs uncrossed. Rest your arm on a flat surface at the level of your heart.

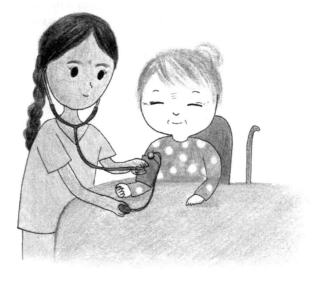

What can I do to reduce my risk?

Some risk factors such as age, race and genetics are out of your control. But there are many lifestyle changes we can make to reduce our risk.

Aim for weight loss if you are overweight. Consume a diet rich in fruits, vegetables, whole grains, low-fat dairy products, and reduced saturated fats. Reduce dietary sodium to less than 1500mg per day. Aim for an intake of dietary potassium of 3500 to 5000mg per day.

Aerobic physical activity of 150 minutes per week. Reduce alcohol consumption to no more than 2 drinks daily for men and 1 drink daily for women. Quit smoking. Manage stress.

Diabetes Mellitus

What is diabetes mellitus?

Diabetes occurs when your blood sugar is too high. Usually, ther pancreas produces insulin to move sugar from the blood into our cells to be stored or used for energy. In people with diabetes, the body does not make enough insulin or is unable to effectively use the insulin. Too much blood sugar can eventually damage our organs, including our heart, kidneys, eyes and nerves.

What are the signs and symptoms of diabetes?

There might not be any symptoms for early diabetes. For some, they might experience increase thirst, hunger, frequent peeing, unexplained weight loss, fatigue, nausea, frequent infections and slow healing cuts or sores.

Am I at risk of getting it?

The exact cause is unknown but we do know certain factors increase the risk:

- Being overweight (body mass index $\geq 23 kg/m^2$)
- Physical inactivity
- Hypertension
- Heart disease
- Hyperlipidaemia
- Family history of diabetes
- Women who had gestational diabetes
- Women with polycystic ovarian disease
- Tuberculosis
- Ethnicity — Indian, Malay, African, Caribbean.

How do I detect it?

You can go for a fasting blood glucose test and glycosylated haemoglobin (HbA1c) if you have any of the risk factors or from age 40 onwards. However, HbA1c is not suitable as choice of test if you have anaemia or thalassaemia.

What can I do to reduce my risk?

Eat more vegetables, fruits, whole grains, fish and low fat dairy products. Avoid food high in saturated fats such as animal fats, full fat dairy products, red meat, egg yolks and palm oil. Exercise for at least 150 minutes per week. Lose weight if you are overweight.

Breast Cancer

What is breast cancer?

Breast cancer occurs when the breast cells become abnormal and begin to grow out of control. Breast cancer remains the most common cancer in women for the past fifty years. There are 6 new cases diagnosed daily and slightly more than 1 death daily.

What are the signs and symptoms of breast cancer?

Most of the time, there are no symptoms in early breast cancer.

If you develop a change in size, shape or appearance of your breast, or notice a lump in your breast or armpit, see a doctor for an assessment. Other symptoms may include bloody discharge from the nipple or a retracted nipple.

Am I at risk of getting it?

All women are at risk.

Our risk in developing breast cancer increases sharply from age 30 and peaks around 60–79 years.

Other risk factors that further increase our risk include:

- Family history of breast cancer
- Early onset of menstruation before the age of 12
- Late menopause after the age of 55
- Not having children
- Late childbearing
- No experience of breastfeeding
- Lack of exercise
- Obesity
- Alcohol consumption
- Being on hormone replacement therapy for a long time.

How do I detect it?

Go for a mammogram every 2 years from age 50 until you are 69 years old. This allows detection of breast cancers before we can physically feel them. These small tumours are likely to be in the early stage and more easily treated.

Discuss with your doctor on the benefits, limitations and risks of starting screening annually for women aged 40 to 49 years old. Up to one quarter of all breast cancers are not detected by mammography in women aged 40–49 years old, compared to one tenth of breast cancers in women aged 50 to 69 years old.

Diagnosis and treatment of breast cancer may be delayed because of a 'normal' mammogram.

Women with high-risk gene mutations or BRCA and history of chest radiation therapy should consider Magnetic Resonance Imaging (MRI) breast screening in addition to mammography. MRI cannot replace mammographic screening as some cancers may manifest as micro-calcifications which may not be shown on MRI.

Women with breasts implants (in particular, diffuse breast free silicon injection augmentation) should have an MRI done in place of a mammogram as the implants can obscure the mammogram images.

What can I do to reduce my risk?

Maintain a healthy weight, exercise regularly, breastfeed, avoid alcohol and smoking, and limit hormone replacement therapy.

Colorectal Cancer

What is colorectal cancer?

Colorectal cancer is cancer developing in the large intestines. Most colorectal cancers begin as small precancerous polyps. They usually grow slowly and do not cause any symptoms till they become large and cancerous. In the period 2013–2017, there were nearly 6 cases diagnosed and more than 2 deaths daily.

What are the signs and symptoms of colorectal cancer?

Unfortunately, early colon cancer usually has no symptoms.

If you experience a change of bowel habits, blood mixed with stools, persistent abdominal discomfort, unexplained weight loss or anaemia, see a doctor for further assessment.

Am I at risk of getting it?

All of us are at risk of colorectal cancer. The risks are increased further if we have the following:

- Personal history of colorectal polyps
- Personal history of inflammatory bowel disease
- Family history of colorectal cancer (Lynch syndrome, familial adenomatous polyposis)
- Diabetes
- Obesity
- Cigarette smoking
- High alcohol intake
- Advanced age
- Diet high in fats and calories, low in fruits and vegetables.

How do I detect it?

For average-risk individuals, screening for colorectal cancer should begin at age 50. The Faecal Immunochemical Test (FIT) is a stool test that can detect a tiny amount of blood even if we cannot see the blood with our naked eyes. The presence of blood can indicate early abnormality in the bowel and your doctor will refer you for a colonoscopy. Cancer can be more effectively treated if it is detected early. The FIT test should be done annually.

Faecal immunochemical test (FIT)-DNA test is an alternative screening test to the FIT stool test. It combines the FIT with detection of abnormal DNA that might be from cancerous polyps in the faeces. You can do the FIT-DNA test once every 3 years if initial screening is normal.

Colonoscopy is the best screening test for colorectal cancer from age 50 onwards. You will be prescribed laxatives to clear your bowels the night before the colonoscopy. The following morning, you will be given light sedation to ease any discomfort while the specialist inserts a colonoscope (a thin tube with light and camera) through the anus to visualise the entire colon. This allows detection and removal of precancerous polyps. You can repeat this procedure every 5–10 years if the initial screening is normal.

Computed Tomography (CT) Colonography is an alternative screening test to a colonoscopy. CT colonography is also known as Virtual Colonoscopy. It uses CT scans to visualise the bowels. No sedation is needed and it is less invasive compared to a colonoscopy as there is no insertion of a colonoscope.

You will be asked to follow a low residue diet and prescribed laxatives the day before the CT scan. You can do this once every 5 years if the initial screening is normal.

If you have 1 or more family members with colorectal cancer, the age to begin screening would be 10 years before the youngest case in the family.

What can I do to reduce my risk?

Maintain a healthy weight. Exercise regularly. Include a diet with emphasis on vegetables, fruits and whole grains. Limit red meat (beef, pork or lamb) and processed meats (sausages, ham or luncheon meat).

Avoid alcohol and quit smoking.

Uterine Cancer

What is uterine cancer?

Uterine cancer is cancer of the womb. It is the fourth most common cancer in women and it is on the upward trend. 70% of the cases occur after age 50.

What are the signs and symptoms of uterine cancer?

Signs and symptoms include abnormal vaginal bleeding, discharge or discomfort. Post-menopausal bleeding is the commonest symptom.

Am I at risk of getting it?

Uterine cancer risk increases from age 30 onwards, peaking at 50–69 years. You are at increased risk if the following factors apply to you:

- Delayed childbearing
- Having few or no children
- Early onset of menstruation
- Late onset of menopause
- Not ovulating regularly, missing menses
- Being on hormone replacement therapy
- Obesity
- Diabetes

- Polycystic ovarian syndrome
- Hereditary nonpolyposis colon cancer or Lynch syndrome
- Tamoxifen.

In up to 40% of uterine cancer cases, no risk factors were identified.

How do I detect it?

A pelvic ultrasound is used to look at the uterus, ovaries and fallopian tubes. It can detect tumours in the uterus or thickened endometrium lining. An endometrial sampling or dilation and curettage can be done by a gynaecologist to diagnose the condition.

What can I do to reduce my risk of getting it?

Maintain a healthy weight and exercise regularly. Discuss with your doctor the pros and cons of being on hormone therapy.

Ovarian Cancer

What is ovarian cancer?

Women have two ovaries. Cancer occurs when ovarian cells grow out of control. We see a rising incidence of ovarian cancer and it is currently the fifth most common cancer in women.

What are the signs and symptoms of ovarian cancer?

There are no early signs or symptoms of ovarian cancer; hence, it is usually discovered in the late stages.

Some women might experience lower abdominal discomfort, bloating, increase in waist size, having to pee more often or change in bowel habits.

Am I at risk of getting it?

Risk factors include:

- Delayed childbearing and having fewer children
- Being on hormone replacement therapy

- Lack of exercise/limited physical activity
- Obesity
- Cigarette smoking
- Age
- Having cancers such as breast cancer, colorectal cancer or uterine cancer
- Family history of ovarian cancer.

How do I detect it?

A pelvic ultrasound as screening for ovarian cancer may be considered.

What factors reduce my risk?

- Pregnancy
- Breastfeeding
- Oral contraceptives provide some protection from ovarian cancer. Protection seems to continue for many years after stopping the pill.
- Sterilisation or hysterectomy (removal of the uterus) may reduce the risk.

Cervical Cancer

What is cervical cancer?

Cervical cancer arises in the neck of the womb. 70 percent of cervical cancer is caused by infection from the human papilloma virus (HPV) subtypes 16 and 18.

Cervical cancer ranking fell from second most common in the 1970s to tenth place between 2008 and 2012. This is largely attributed to the start of country-wide pap smear screening and early treatment of pre-invasive cervical cancer.

What are the signs and symptoms of cervical cancer?

Signs and symptoms include abnormal vaginal bleeding, discharge, pain during sexual intercourse, painful urination, leaking of urine or stools from the vagina.

Am I at risk of getting it?

Your risk is increased if you have multiple sexual partners or had unprotected sex from a young age.

How do I detect it?

All women who have ever had sexual intercourse should undergo cervical cancer screening from age 25. Women aged 25 to 29 should be screened with the pap smear, at least once every 3 years. A pap smear can detect abnormal cells.

Women aged 30 years and above should be screened with HPV testing once every 5 years. If you screen positive for the 16 or 18 HPV strains, you should see a gynaecologist for a colposcopy test.

What can I do to reduce my risk?

Human papillomavirus (HPV) vaccination has been included in the National Childhood and Adult Immunisation Schedule. Started in 2019, MOH introduced free HPV vaccination to Secondary One female students. It is most effective if given before the first experience of sexual intercourse.

Women who are sexually active may still benefit from the vaccine as they may not have been exposed to the types of HPV covered by the vaccine.

Further Reading

50 Years of Cancer Registration. Singapore Cancer Registry. Available at: https://www.nrdo.gov.sg/docs/librariesprovider3/default-document-library/thespore-cancerregistry_commerativebook_-1.pdf?sfvrsn= 231fce6e_0.

Arnett DK, Blumenthal RS, Albert MA, *et al.* 2019 ACC/AHA guideline on the primary prevention of cardiovascular disease: executive summary. A report of the ACC/AHA taskforce on clinical practice guidelines. *J Am Coll Cardiol* 2019; 74(10): 1376–1414.

Conditions and Treatments and Medicines. SingHealth. Available at: https://www.singhealth.com.sg/patient-care/conditions-treatments.

Glossary of Local Health Topics: Diseases and Conditions. Health Hub. Available at: https://www.healthhub.sg/a-z/a?cat=diseases-and-conditions.

Kaur A. Cardiovascular Disease the Leading Cause of Death for Women in Singapore Last Year. *Straits Times;* 2020 Oct 4. Available at: https://www.straitstimes.com/lifestyle/cardiovascular-disease-the-leading-cause-of-death-for-women-in-singapore-last-year.

Report of the Screening Test Review Committee. Academy of Medicine, Singapore; 2019 Mar. Available at: https://www.ams.edu.sg/view-pdf.aspx?file=media%5c4817_fi_59.pdf&ofile=STRC+Report+March+2019.pdf.

BREAST CANCER

Take Home Points

1. Adopt healthy lifestyle habits.
2. Do your own breast self-examination once your breasts develop.
3. See a doctor to start mammogram screening from age 40.
4. Speak to a doctor if you have any concerns, do not self-diagnose from internet sites.
5. When detected early, breast cancer can be treated, and we can resume a normal life afterwards.

How do I look after my breast?

1. All women can start doing their own breast self-examination on a monthly basis, once breasts develop.
2. Starting from age 40, one can start doing yearly mammograms, and add on ultrasound if one has dense breasts.
3. If you detect a lump, please consult a doctor early. While not all lumps are cancerous, early detection of cancer saves lives.

Dr Tan Yia Swam is a General Surgeon, specializing in Breast cancer care and treatment, and is the founder of Breast Friend Surgery & Wellness, and Clinical Director of Thomson Breast Centre. She is also a visiting Consultant at Nexus Surgical group.

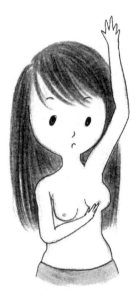

How do I do a breast self-examination?

1. Try to do it in the shower — it's convenient, there's probably a mirror, and it's easier to feel for lumps with a bit of soapy water.
2. Put your hands on your hips and look out for changes in breast shape, skin surface, and nipple abnormalities. Raise the left arm above your head to look for changes (especially dimples) on the skin of the left breast. Use two to three fingers from your right hand to press into the breast tissue, in a systematic manner. Repeat this step on the right breast.
3. Start from the top (12 o'clock area), press down and massage in a circular manner, gradually move around the breast to cover all areas, and from outside in, towards the nipple.
4. Last step, squeeze the nipple gently to check for nipple discharge. Then repeat on the right breast.

You should look out for painless lumps, unusual nipple discharge (e.g., bloody/greenish/yellowish fluid that is not milk), retracted nipples, persistent rash around the nipple, dimpled and puckered skin, or swollen and thickened skin.

Normal breast tissue has a lumpy quality to it, and depending on how much body fat one has, or the timing of menses, sometimes the lumpiness may feel more obvious, and more sensitive.

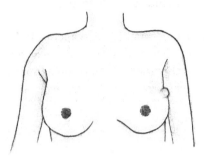

Some important facts to share:

1. Breast pain alone is not a symptom of cancer.
2. Most cancers are found by chance on screening mammograms, or ultrasound scans.
3. Some women with breast cancer may have a lump, or nipple discharge.
4. Most lumps are not cancerous. Your doctor will use a combination of history taking (to know your risk factors), relevant imaging (mammogram and ultrasound), and maybe a biopsy (needle test) to diagnose what you have.
5. All breast cancers can be treated; the stage will affect the prognosis.

I have an abnormal mammogram: what happens next?

Mammograms (MMG) are X-rays of the breast, and help to detect early breast cancer.

The breast contains glands, milk ducts, fat, and fibrous tissue, all under the skin.

On an X-ray, the glandular tissue will be 'dense', meaning it looks white and thus may cover up small lumps, or calcium spots.

There are several types of abnormalities:

1. Dense breast: which is a common variant. Speak to your doctor for any need to do additional, supplementary scans.

2. Opacity: this means a shadow, which might be a lump, or sometimes just overlapping tissue.
3. Microcalcifications: These are calcium deposits.
4. Others: stromal/architectural distortions.

Note that not all abnormalities are cancers. In fact, the majority of these abnormalities will turn out to be normal. If you go for a routine mammogram and your doctor says that there could be an abnormality, you would usually be referred to a breast surgeon for further evaluation.

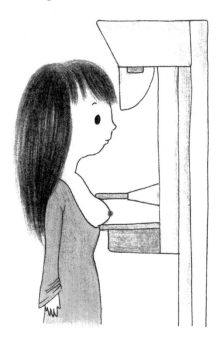

I have an abnormal ultrasound of the breasts, what should I do?

An ultrasound (US) uses sound waves to study tissue, and this same technology is used to scan a baby's growth during pregnancy. In the breast area, doctors usually recommend it as an add on scan for women whose mammogram images indicate dense breasts, or when the woman complains of a symptom such as a lump, or nipple discharge.

Most specialists would not recommend breast US screening in a well, asymptomatic woman. However, it is commonly offered in many health packages. There are many small non-cancerous lumps in the breast (cysts, fibroadenomas), which are small, less than 1cm, so they cannot be felt. These are not harmful. If a well, asymptomatic woman never has an ultrasound done, she would not be aware of such lumps, and thus not suffer any consequences. However, once a US is done and picks up many small lumps (also called nodules), most women react with worry or even panic, as they think that the nodules are all cancerous.

Hence, if you have an ultrasound done, and your doctor explains that it is abnormal, you would usually be referred to a breast specialist to discuss the next steps, otherwise, there is no cause for worry.

Some common scenarios:

1. The lumps clearly look benign — leave them alone.
2. The lumps should be benign, but it would be good to continue monitoring them on a yearly basis.
3. The lumps look indeterminate (e.g., too small to tell if they are benign or cancerous) — the options are monitoring closely every 6 months, or doing a biopsy to be sure.

When are biopsies done?

After the breast surgeon speaks to the patient, examines and reviews the MMG/US images, a biopsy may be recommended. For findings where it is indeterminate (i.e., 30–60 percent chance of cancer), or suspicious (>80 percent chance of cancer), a core needle biopsy will help in diagnosis.

This is usually done as a clinic procedure, or as day surgery, under local anaesthetic. It may be done with mammogram or ultrasound guidance, depending on how the abnormality was detected. The abnormality (whether microcalcifications, or lump) is sampled a few times, through a small (2–3mm cut). The samples are then sent to the lab for analysis.

The lab results are usually ready in 3–7 working days, depending on whether additional special tests are needed. Results are broadly divided into three groups:

1. Benign — in which case your doctor may recommend that it's ok to just monitor the area, or you could request for a minor surgery to remove it once and for all.

2. Atypia — this means that there are abnormal cells, which are not cancerous yet, but need removal, as they might develop into cancer.
3. Cancer — this might be DCIS (ductal carcinoma in situ), or invasive cancer.

I have been diagnosed with breast cancer — what happens now?

If your biopsy showed cancer, your doctor would need to explain to you whether it is a DCIS, or invasive cancer.

DCIS, is also called 'stage zero' cancer, as this indicates cancerous changes. DCIS does not spread to other areas. As such, most patients may just need surgery, and maybe radiotherapy or hormonal tablets. Chemotherapy is not needed. Patients with DCIS have excellent prognosis (i.e., More than 95 percent may be cancer free even after 20 years).

If it is an invasive cancer, your doctor would likely arrange for a whole body scan to check if there is any spread to other organs. Additional lab tests may be performed on the biopsy specimens (ER/PR/her2). These indicate the type of breast cancer, how sensitive they are to female hormones, or how likely they are to keep growing.

With this information, your surgeon may send you to a chemo doctor (medical oncologist) to discuss the pros and cons of the various combinations of treatment:

1. Surgery first, followed by chemotherapy, maybe radiotherapy, or hormonal tablets.
2. Chemotherapy first, followed by surgery, maybe radiotherapy, or hormonal tablets.

There have been many advances in the past 10 years, in surgical techniques, and types of chemotherapy. If you have cancer, do discuss with your doctors to find out what is best for you.

The treatments will take up to one year to complete. Subsequently, cancer basis patients will be on regular follow-up, on a 3-monthly, or 6-monthly basis, for up to 5 years, or even longer.

DIABETES

Take Home Points

1. Diabetes can be a silent disease, most cases are only diagnosed when screening blood tests are done.
2. Pre-diabetes can progress to Type 2 diabetes, but can also return to normal with strict lifestyle and diet changes.
3. Gestational diabetes in pregnancy can affect the pregnancy's outcome and affect the health of the baby, hence it is important to have good glucose control if you are diagnosed with gestational diabetes.
4. Complications of diabetes include damage to the kidney, eyes and nerves, as well as blockage of important arteries which can lead to strokes, heart attacks and poor circulation to the feet. These can be avoided if diabetes is well controlled.
5. There is a wide variety of medications which can be used to control blood sugar. You can discuss with your doctor which medications are most suitable for you.

Dr Tay Tunn Lin is a Consultant Endocrinologist, specializing in Diabetes, with special interest in young adults with diabetes, and is currently practising at Mount Alvernia Hospital, Mount Elizabeth Orchard, and Parkway East Hospital.

Jane is a 39-year-old woman who is married with 2 children, ages 8 and 6. She works as a marketing executive and feels relatively healthy despite putting on about 8 kg gradually since the birth of her last child. She had been busy looking after her children and with her work, she hardly had time to exercise. "Weight gain is inevitable after having kids and when metabolism slows down," she thought.

However, she had a rude shock after she underwent an employee health screening offered by her company — her results came back with the diagnosis of diabetes. She had not felt unwell at all and she was still relatively young.

These are some of the questions that she has about diabetes.

What is diabetes?

Diabetes is a chronic medical condition where the blood glucose (or sugar) levels are too high. When the blood glucose levels are always high for long periods of time, this can lead to multiple health problems. Hence, diabetes needs to be aggressively tackled; the aim is to keep the blood glucose within its normal range.

Insulin is a hormone that is produced by our body; it allows glucose from the food we eat to be absorbed and used as energy. It is like a key which 'unlocks' the doors to our cells to allow glucose to enter and be used by the cells of our body.

When there is insufficient insulin being produced or if the body is unable to use the insulin, glucose is unable to enter our body's cells and hence blood glucose levels remain high. When the body is unable to use the insulin, this is known as 'insulin resistance' — this means that high levels of insulin is being produced, but our cells refuse to allow insulin to work. This usually occurs in the more commonly diagnosed Type 2 diabetes.

In Singapore, we have seen a sharp rise in our population being diagnosed with diabetes from 2004 to 2010 in both males and females, with a higher prevalence in men than women, but with greater severity in women. Pre-menopausal women with diabetes lose the protection against heart disease that non-diabetic women have and are 50 percent more likely to die from heart disease than men. Cyclical hormonal changes make diabetes control more difficult in pre-menopausal women. There are also issues of high glucose levels during pregnancy, affecting not just the mother, but also the baby. Elderly post-menopausal women who have kidney failure are at a higher risk of dying than men with a similar problem.

Table 1. Crude prevalence of diabetes (%) among Singapore residents aged 18 to 69 years.

Year	1998	2004	2010
Total	9.0	8.2	11.3
Age group			
18–29	0.8	0.5	1.0
30–39	3.3	2.4	4.3
40–49	9.6	7.9	12.1
50–59	21.8	16.7	19.3
60–69	32.4	28.7	29.1
Gender			
Male	8.5	8.9	12.3
Female	9.6	7.6	10.4

Source: National Health Survey 1998, 2004, 2010, Ministry of Health, Singapore.

Does eating too much sugary food cause diabetes?

Diet alone is not responsible for diabetes. There is a genetic and lifestyle component to Type 2 diabetes, which is a combination of deficiency of insulin release and insulin resistance. Insulin resistance results from excessive body weight and belly fat. This causes the body to fight back by producing more insulin from the pancreas. Over time, the demand for more insulin outpaces the ability of the pancreas to produce it, leading to the development of pre-diabetes or diabetes.

This is different from Type 1 diabetes, which is irrespective of our body shape. Type 1 diabetes arises from our body's immune system attacking the pancreas cells that produces insulin. Once antibodies are triggered to attack the pancreatic cells, insulin production is impaired, and this leads to absolute insulin deficiency.

Sugary foods contribute to weight gain, which can worsen insulin resistance and hasten the progression to diabetes. Hence to prevent diabetes, it is advisable to stay away from a diet filled with excessive sugar. The maximum amount of added sugar limit per day for a woman is about 7 teaspoons (25g) and for a man, it is about 9 teaspoons (35g). A can of soda or soft drink has about 8 teaspoons of sugar, which means that makes up the entire day's quota![1]

Can diabetes be cured?

Diabetes is a chronic condition which does not go away after a period of time, unlike the flu. But it can be managed by ensuring the blood glucose levels remain within the acceptable range to prevent complications from occurring. The complications are widespread across various organ systems.

Diabetes cannot be cured but can be controlled. Some patients with mild diabetes may be able to come off medications after improving their diet, lifestyle and losing weight. If these interventions are not maintained, their glucose can still go up again. Hence, they are not considered 'cured' but in remission.

Results from a 2018 study indicated that 50 percent of participants (with an average BMI above 27 kg/m^2) were able to lose an average of 10 kg through intensive dietary interventions and also achieve remission of their diabetes.[2]

Jane recalled that during her second pregnancy, she had some blood tests done which showed that she had high glucose levels, but this was controlled by her cutting back on food high in sugar. After delivery, she was told she did not have diabetes.

Why were her glucose levels high during pregnancy yet normalised later? Was this a factor in her current diagnosis of diabetes?

Diabetes can be classified into:

a.   Pre-diabetes
b.   Type 2 diabetes
c.   Type 1 diabetes
d.   Gestational diabetes

What Jane had was gestational diabetes — a condition where high glucose levels occurs only during pregnancy. The multiple hormonal changes causes insulin resistance which prevents the body from producing sufficient insulin. In such patients, there is no pre-existing condition of diabetes before pregnancy; this high glucose levels only occurs during pregnancy. Up to 1 in 5 pregnant ladies in Singapore have gestational diabetes.

In Singapore, pregnant patients undergo screening for gestational diabetes with an oral glucose tolerance test towards the end of the second trimester of pregnancy. This involves a fasting blood test, drinking a sugary drink that contains 75g of glucose, then drawing blood to check the glucose levels again 1h and 2h after.

High glucose levels can cause complications in the baby, such as causing it to grow too large, leading to a difficult delivery with potential damage to the baby's nerves in the neck or arm; breathing difficulties in the baby after delivery; low blood sugar levels leading to seizures in the baby; and even still birth. The child also has an increased risk of obesity and diabetes in future.

How is gestational diabetes treated?

Gestational diabetes requires strict dietary control during pregnancy. Dieticians would advise on how to achieve glucose control without compromising nutritional requirements. If diet alone is insufficient to control glucose, medications such as insulin will have to be started so that pregnancy outcomes are optimised. The typical glucose targets during pregnancy are much stricter than non-pregnant states, and finger prick glucose readings are needed up to 7 times a day, pre-meals and 2 hours post-meals. Pre-meal targets should be <5.3 mmol/L and 2-hour post-meal targets are <6.7 mmol/L. The aim is to get glucose readings as near to normal as possible to provide the best environment for the developing baby.

The good news is, that this condition usually goes away after delivery, when the hormonal changes in pregnancy have returned to normal and thus reduced insulin resistance. But screening for diabetes should still be done after delivery as up to 40% may go on to have pre-diabetes within 5 years.

What is pre-diabetes?

Pre-diabetes, as its name suggests, is a condition where the criteria for overt diabetes has not been fulfilled, but represents part of the spectrum that is somewhere in between what is normal and what is considered to be diabetes. There is evidence that pre-diabetes can progress to diabetes in up to 74 percent of people within 10 years. Interestingly, men have pre-diabetes for an average of 8.5 years and women for 10.3 years before they develop diabetes.[3]

Pre-diabetes is also not as benign as one may think. It can increase the risk of heart disease, stroke and deaths by up to 30 percent.[4] It is postulated that women have to undergo greater deterioration of their metabolic complications before they develop diabetes, compared to men. This means that women have worse levels of cholesterol and higher blood pressure before they progress from pre-diabetes to diabetes. Having multiple risk factors like hypertension, high cholesterol and diabetes increases the chances of getting heart disease and stroke. Because of the concomitant other risk factors that are associated with pre-diabetes in women, they have a higher risk of heart disease and stroke compared to men.[3]

How is pre-diabetes treated?

A person with pre-diabetes can actually return to having normal glucose tolerance. The best way to achieve this is through lifestyle improvement. It is proven in robust studies that healthy diets, exercising and losing weight when we are overweight can reduce progression to diabetes by 37 percent over 6 years. This includes maintaining a BMI that is <23 or in those who are overweight, losing about 5 to 10 percent of their baseline weight.

There are medications that can be started, but only after lifestyle changes have been made. These include metformin or acarbose tablets. Medications reduce disease progression by 26 percent while intensive lifestyle changes reduces disease progression by 37 percent.

Now that Jane has been diagnosed with diabetes, how can it be treated?

The management of diabetes consists of 3 pillars: diet, exercise and medication.

Diet

Having a healthy diet is the cornerstone of diabetes management. Foods which raise blood glucose levels are carbohydrates and those with added sugar, such as chocolates, candies, donuts and sweetened beverages. Carbohydrates include not just white rice, but noodles, bread, pasta, potatoes and chapati as well. Carbohydrates should not be totally excluded from our meals but we need to be mindful of the portions of carbohydrates that we eat. Following the diagnosis of diabetes, it is advisable for patients to consult a dietician to find out what is an appropriate amount of carbohydrates for their individual age, weight, and activity level.[5]

There are many different types of diet plans that have been popularised by celebrities to help with weight loss and even diabetes. These include the keto diet, Mediterranean diet, paleo diet, vegan diet and intermittent fasting.

Is there evidence that these diets will improve health?

The most robust research available related to eating patterns for pre-diabetes or Type 2 diabetes prevention are Mediterranean-style, low-fat, or low carbohydrate eating plans. In particular, the Mediterranean style diet was examined in patients over a period of 4 years in the PREDIMED study — diabetes control improved with a decrease in the number of medications needed. There was also a decrease in heart disease in the patients on this diet.[6]

Another popular diet pattern is intermittent fasting. There are different approaches to this: time-restricted eating to only 8 hours within the day or alternate day fasting with restriction of calories etc. The studies done are small and of short duration. Still, they demonstrated that within the intervention group, there was significant weight loss, improved insulin sensitivity, improved insulin production, improvements in blood pressure, oxidative stress, and appetite.

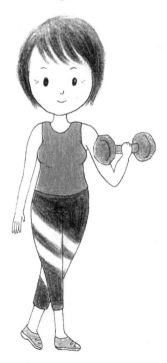

Exercise

For many women, weight gain can be traced back to the time around pregnancy. It is difficult for most to shed the pounds after pregnancy. Juggling motherhood and a career can also mean one has less time for exercise. For others, weight may have been a struggle since they were young and a problem for other family members as well, suggesting that genes play a role.

Exercise has benefits on our metabolic health. It helps to lower blood pressure, lower harmful LDL cholesterol and triglycerides, raise healthy HDL cholesterol, strengthen muscles and bones, lower glucose levels, boost our sensitivity to insulin and counter insulin resistance. It also helps to relieve stress, reduce anxiety and improve our overall well-being.

It doesn't matter what type of exercise we do, aerobic or resistance; they are both equally good at lowering glucose in people with diabetes. It was found that women with diabetes who exercise 3–4 hours a week, had a 40 percent lower risk of getting heart disease than those who did not. This averages to exercising 30 minutes daily.

In patients who are on insulin, it is important to check their blood glucose with a finger prick reading before exercising as the glucose level will decrease such that it can lead to hypoglycaemia (where blood glucose levels are too low causing tremors, sweating and hunger pangs) during or after the exercise. If the glucose reading is below 5.5 mmol/L, it may be prudent to eat a fruit, like a banana or 2–3 pieces of plain crackers before exercising.

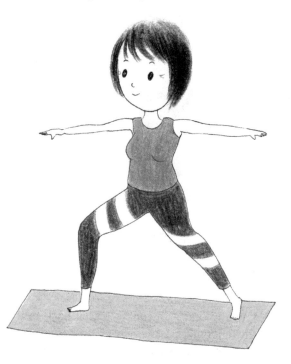

Medication

Anti-diabetic medications are very helpful in managing glucose levels and keeping the readings within the body's normal range.

These can be oral therapy or injectable therapies. Both have their roles in the treatment of diabetes.

(a) Oral medications for Type 2 diabetes:

Metformin: This is a medication that works by reducing liver production of glucose and improving the sensitivity of the body to insulin. It also reduces the amount of sugar being absorbed from the foods we eat. It has been used and studied extensively for many years and is very safe and effective. The minor side effects commonly experienced would be diarrhoea, nausea or abdominal gassiness initially, but it is typically well tolerated if the dose is increased gradually over time.

Sulfonylurea: There are many types of sulfonylureas and this class of medication works by increasing the release of insulin from our pancreas. It is effective in lowering blood sugar levels but should be taken only if regular meals are taken, to avoid the side effect of hypoglycemia. It can also cause mild weight gain and increased appetite. Examples of these medications include gliclazide, glipizide, tolbutamide.

Dipeptidyl peptidase 4 inhibitor (DPP4 inhibitors): There are several types of DPP4 inhibitors and all had been tested in large studies which had proven their safety and effectiveness in the treatment of Type 2 diabetes. It works by stopping the breakdown of the dipeptidyl peptidase enzyme which increases the levels of incretin hormones, which in turn, increases release of insulin when glucose levels are high, to control glucose levels. Examples of these medications include linagliptin, saxagliptin, sitagliptin.

Sodium-glucose co-transporter 2 inhibitor (SGLT2i): This class of medication works on the kidneys which stops the reabsorption of glucose by the kidneys, allowing more glucose to be excreted via the urine, in the range of 60–100g loss of glucose per day. Besides lowering blood glucose to achieve better diabetes control, with the loss of calories from the urine, it also helps to lower body weight, and blood pressure. Recent studies done also found that it helps to protect against heart failure, reduces the risk of deaths related to heart disease and kidney protection effects. Side effects include increase in risk of infections in the groin or urinary tract infections, mild dehydration and excessive keto-acids in the blood in patients who are fasting yet continue to take the medication. It is advisable to consult your doctor if you are on a keto diet or are scheduled for surgery that requires prolonged fasting; check whether you can have the medication stopped temporarily. Examples of this medication includes empagliflozin, dapagliflozin, canagliflozin.

Alpha glucosidase inhibitor: Acarbose belongs to this family of medications called alpha glucosidase inhibitor. It works by slowing down an enzyme in the intestine which breaks down food into sugars in the gut, leading to a slower rate of absorption of glucose into our blood. Potentially, it can also improve insulin resistance. Its side effect includes increase abdominal gassiness, diarrhoea and, less commonly, abnormality in liver blood test.

(b) Injectable therapies:

Glucagon-like peptide 1 receptor antagonist (GLP1RA) for Type 2 diabetes: Patients with Type 2 diabetes do not make sufficient GLP1 hormones which are released from the intestines after eating to reduce blood glucose levels and signal to our brain that we are full. GLP1RA injections, which range from weekly to daily injections, are highly effective in lowering blood glucose and also helps to control appetite. Many patients can lose up to 5 to 10 percent of their baseline weight! It has also been found to be protective of the heart and reduce cardiovascular deaths and stroke in patients with diabetes. Examples of GLP1RA include liraglutide, exenatide, dulaglutide.

Insulin: Insulin is still the mainstay of treatment in patients with Type 1 diabetes, advanced Type 2 diabetes, and poorly controlled diabetes. Insulin goes back a long way in history, but technology has advanced greatly and now, insulin is much more purified, with a function that more closely mimics our bodies' own insulin actions. Insulin is still mainly an injectable medication. Depending on the type, some patients may just need injections once a day whilst others may need them up to 4 times a day. It can be used concurrently with oral diabetes medications, depending on the individual's condition.

Also, insulin can be used in insulin pumps which are portable machines that allow better fine-tuning of how insulin is delivered to the body on a minute-to-minute basis — this requires patients to be invested in learning how to use the pump and to adjust how much insulin is given for meals and activities with very frequent glucose monitoring.

Jane is worried because she has heard that diabetes can lead to complications like kidney failure. She wonders what other complications diabetes can cause.

Diabetes complications can be broadly categorised into 2 main groups:

1. Microvascular complications (complications related to small blood vessels in the body)
   - Eyes
   - Kidneys
   - Nerves
2. Macrovascular complications (complications related to large blood vessels in the body)
   - Heart disease
   - Stroke
   - Gangrene of the foot

In the eyes, damage to the blood vessels and retina (known as diabetic retinopathy) can lead to blindness over time without any preceding symptoms. Only with screening can early diabetic eye changes be detected; thus, doctors will schedule patients with diabetes for yearly eye screening. This involves using a specialized machine to take a photo of the retina or using an ophthalmoscope which shines a bright light into the eyes to allow examination of the retina.

Another microvascular complication is in the kidneys. High blood glucose levels affect the arteries in the body. The kidneys filter blood from those arteries. Up to 40 percent of patients with diabetes develop some kind of kidney disease. Stress to the kidneys lead to leakage of protein through the urine, or difficulty in clearing waste effectively from the body, or the inability to maintain normal fluid balance in the body.

Diabetes-related kidney disease is the most common cause of kidney failure in the world. Poorly controlled diabetes and high blood pressure are important risk factors for kidney damage. Early kidney damage is asymptomatic but can be detected many years before end stage renal failure.

Early detection gives one time to have better control of diabetes, blood pressure and cholesterol to prevent progression of the condition. It is screened for yearly through blood and urine tests. If symptomatic, it may indicate advanced kidney failure. Symptoms include swelling of the feet, breathlessness on lying flat or upon exertion, vomiting and nausea.

The last microvascular (small blood vessel) complication is peripheral neuropathy, where diabetes affects the nerves of the hands and feet. Typical symptoms include numbness of the hands or feet or a tingly, painful sensation which can affect sleep. This loss of sensation can lead to undetected foot ulcers from even minor trauma which can lead to infections. For example, a blister from a new pair of shoes can easily develop into a poor healing wound which gets infected. The infection can be so severe that it leads to amputation of part of the foot. As part of diabetes management, just like how screening is done for the eyes and the kidneys, screening is also done for peripheral neuropathy by using the monofilament test.

What are the macrovascular complications?

In the heart, there can be buildup of plaque which leads to a narrowing of the blood vessels supplying blood to the heart. When blood flow to the heart is diminished, it can cause blockages and heart attacks.

In the brain, the same process of plaque buildup in the arteries (a type of blood vessel) can lead to decreased blood flow. When the blood vessel is completely blocked, a stroke can occur.

Diabetes can affect the blood vessels of the feet, leading to poor blood circulation. This, together with the neuropathy, leads to poor healing wounds, which can get infected or develop into gangrene (dead, infected tissue), requiring an amputation. Blockage of the arteries to the feet can lead to gangrene. Some patients have both neuropathy and poor circulation which leads to feet ulcers that do not heal.

Nevertheless, it is not all downhill after receiving a diagnosis of diabetes. Controlling diabetes, together with blood pressure and cholesterol can help prevent the onset and progression of these complications. This is especially important during the first 1 to 2 years of diagnosis. Good control during the early phases of diabetes has a much greater impact in preventing diabetes complications. However, it will still make a difference at any point of the disease.

Jane now has a clearer idea of what diabetes is. She knows that she has control over her health — by changing her diet and lifestyle, being compliant to her medications and going for regular check-ups — all of these will help her reach her goal of staying healthy for years to come.

Further Reading

Estruch R, Ros E, Salas-Salvadó J, *et al.* Primary prevention of cardiovascular disease with a mediterranean diet supplemented with extra-virgin olive oil or nuts. *N Engl J Med* 2018; 378: e34.

Evert AB, Dennison M, Gardner CD, *et al.* Nutrition therapy for adults with diabetes or prediabetes: a consensus report. *Diabetes Care* 2019 May; 42(5): 731–754.

How Much Sugar is Too Much? American Heart Association. Available at: https://www.heart.org/en/healthy-living/healthy-eating/eat-smart/sugar/how-much-sugar-is-too-much.

Huang Y, Cai X, Mai W, *et al.* Association between prediabetes and risk of cardiovascular disease and all cause ortality: systematic review and meta-analysis. *BMJ* 2016; 355: i5953. doi: 10.1136/bmj.i5953.

JWJ, Rutters F, Ryden L, *et al.* Risk and management of pre-diabetes. *Eur J Prev Cardiol* 2019 Dec; 26(2S): 47–54. doi: 10.1177/2047487319880041.

Lean MEJ, Leslie WS, Barnes AC, *et al.* Primary care-led weight management for remission of type 2 diabetes (DiRECT): an open-label, cluster-randomised trial *Lancet* 2018 Feb; 391(10120): 541–551. doi: 10.1016/S0140-6736(17)33102-1.

ISCHAEMIC HEART DISEASE

Take Home Points

1. The risk of heart attack in women shows a marked increase after menopause.
2. Early diagnosis and treatment of hypertension, diabetes and hypercholesterolemia is key to the prevention of heart disease.
3. Symptoms may be non-specific in females and easily missed, so regular health screening is important.
4. Prevention is better than cure. A healthy lifestyle with a good diet, sufficient sleep and moderate exercise is important for heart health.
5. Taking appropriate medications as prescribed by the cardiologists may be life-saving.

Symptoms of Heart Disease

The cardinal symptoms of heart disease are chest pain, palpitations and shortness of breath. Listed below are some common complaints and how best to deal with them.

Dr Lim Ing Haan is an Interventional Cardiologist, and is currently practising at Lim Ing Haan Cardiology Clinic in Mount Elizabeth Hospital.

Why do young women get chest pains?

Chest pains are a common complaint. However, the causes of chest pains are vastly different depending on the age of the affected. I shall first describe some of the possible causes in a young working female.

In the younger age group, chest pain most commonly arises from the bones or muscles. This may be due to a condition that typically affects young females called costochondritis, swelling of the joint at the front of the ribs. In fact, pain can be pinpointed to a specific spot on the ribcage. Usually, this is worse when coughing and may be bad enough to affect sleep, but it is easily treated with pain relief.

The other common cause of chest pain in young people is reflux esophagitis or gastritis which causes pain when acid flows back into the oesophagus. A giveaway clue is excessive burping or bloating of the stomach. Pain is made worse by a meal.

The medical term for heart-related pain is angina and that usually comes with other tell-tale symptoms, including a gripping sensation at the throat, or radiation of the pain to the left arm. Together with breathlessness or wild beating of the heart, these may signal a heart attack. Though extremely unlikely in young females, I have treated a young female aged 26 who was admitted to hospital for a heart attack. She was a heavy smoker and a heavy drinker, these factors, coupled with work stress was too much for her! Heart attack is very uncommon in adults younger than 30 but it is by no means unheard of.

Fortunately, young women in the child bearing age group are naturally protected from heart attacks, thanks to the abundance of the female hormones. It is uncommon for women to suffer heart attacks in this age group unless they smoke. So, my advice to young females is to never start smoking. The most common reasons for chest pain is musculoskeletal pain from the joints in the ribs and reflux gastritis. Thus, a trial of antacids may be useful before heading down to the doctor's office.

What is the most common cause of chest pain in post-menopausal females?

Heart disease is the leading cause of death worldwide. Understandably, the risks faced by women depend on the age and presence of risk factors.

Post menopause, there is increased likelihood of artery blockages both in the main arteries and in micro vessels. Chest pains, chest tightness and palpitations should be taken seriously. This is especially so if there is high blood pressure, high cholesterol, diabetes or smoking.

Did you know, women are less likely to be offered standard tests? Studies have shown that routinely in the emergency department, women receive fewer tests compared to men and suffer more from undertreatment when presenting with chest pain. Important tests like the exercise stress test, CT coronary angiogram or cardiac catheterisation should be done whenever there is suspicion of heart disease, accompanied by risk factors.

By the age of 70, the rate of heart disease in women catches up with that of men. So women at this age and above must not ignore chest pains, because globally, as mentioned, women are consistently being underdiagnosed and undertreated for serious heart conditions compared to men. Most importantly, even if the main heart arteries are normal, disease in the micro vessels which cannot be seen, also requires medication as microvascular disease can still cause heart attacks.

Sharp tearing chest pain

Sharp tearing pain with simultaneous cold sweats and difficulty breathing may signal a serious condition known as arterial dissection. It requires immediate medical attention as it represents a tear in the wall of either the aorta or the heart arteries and can be life threatening. Treatment cannot be delayed.

My heart rhythm is irregular and I have difficulty breathing

Another common complaint in middle-aged female is the feeling of palpitations and breathlessness. These complaints are frequently due to heart artery blockages or microvascular disease. During evaluation, we always ask for recent fever or flu first because a recent viral infection can temporarily cause extra heart beats. Thyroid hormone imbalances may also be the culprit. Very uncommonly, gastric reflux may be the actual cause of these symptoms. So, a visit to a doctor, blood tests and ECG are the basic tests required to find out the root cause and to determine if it is a more serious issue requiring a visit to the cardiologist.

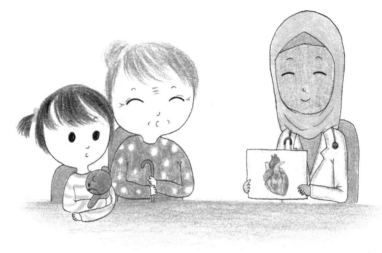

I am breathless, is it normal?

Shortness of breath can be a subjective symptom of lack of fitness and exercise. It is a reflection of the heart or lung function. A rough guide of normality is the ability to walk up 2 flights of stairs or across one block of flats. A common complaint is the difficulty of negotiating a usual activity like going to the market and returning with a load of groceries. This usually highlights the need to undergo a check-up to look for artery blockages.

A weak heart leads to heart failure and breathlessness. Water retention inevitably accumulates in the lungs and causes difficulty breathing, initially noticeable while walking and then progressively noticeable even at rest. When water retention is very advanced and the lungs are congested with fluids, the afflicted is unable to lie flat and may have to rest in a propped up, in a semi-inclined position, commonly awaking a few times at night to cough up pink frothy sputum.

Further escalation of water retention then affects the liver, leading to inability to eat and digest, resulting in a bloated abdomen. At this point, leg swelling progressively worsen and extends up to the knees.

In other words, pay attention to symptoms of breathlessness, inability to lie flat comfortably, coughing at night and leg swelling. These are early signs of heart failure.

Who is at Risk?

Patients are divided into high, moderate or low risk groups. High risk patients are those who have already suffered a heart attack or stroke in the past year. Moderate risks patients are those who have high blood pressure, high levels of bad cholesterol or diabetes. Smoking and obesity are lifestyle factors that increase risks. Advanced age, menopause and a family history of heart attacks and strokes are non-modifiable risk factors. Risks of heart attacks can be modified by lowering cholesterol levels, controlling blood pressure and diabetes. The absolute benefit is greatest in those with high and moderate risks. So, understand your risk to help you decide when to go for health screening.

Investigations

When should I go for screening?

While some people may show signs of an impending heart attack, others may suffer without any symptoms.

With our lifestyles becoming increasingly stressful and sedentary, heart disease is the leading cause of death globally and is projected to remain so. It could also be a silent killer in apparently healthy people who are asymptomatic.

Warning symptoms can be very confusing so rather than being forced to rush to the hospital suddenly, preventive yearly screening is advisable.

Screening is recommended for asymptomatic men aged 45 to 75 years, and asymptomatic women aged 55 to 75 years. Identification of early atherosclerosis (a condition where the artery wall thickens due to the accumulation of fatty substances like cholesterol) helps motivate individuals to take preventive measures. Thus, early screening for heart disease should go beyond basic screening for high blood pressure, high cholesterol, diabetes and obesity. It should include screening for atherosclerosis of the heart and neck arteries.

The main idea is to treat the disease itself and not just the risk factors. Also, those with no evidence of atherosclerosis can be reassured, whereas those with atherosclerosis can be selectively targeted to prevent a heart attack or stroke. There is good evidence that undergoing a Computed Tomography (CT) Scan, measuring the coronary calcium score, or going through a carotid ultrasound can help identify those with high risk of cardiovascular disease.

The main problem that we physicians face is that these tests may identify heart diseases but may not influence behaviour. The physician can help with the diagnosis and prescription of appropriate treatment but the key to compliance to treatment rests entirely in the patient's hands.

ECG — Electrocardiogram

This is a simple test and is available in most clinics. It is performed either routinely or when there is complaint of chest pain to diagnose heart disease and problems of heart rhythm. It important to remember that though ECG cannot predict future heart attacks, routine yearly ECGs has identified heart disease in some patients who do not have symptoms. We usually recommend yearly ECG as part of health screening.

Echocardiogram

2D or 3D Echocardiogram is a specialised ultrasound examination of the heart. Echo is safe and performed without injection or radiation to the patient. It gives important information on the size, structure and function of the heart. This is how we can diagnose cases of enlarged heart, weak heart, or diseases of the heart valves. If heart function is weak, further tests to look for blockage of the coronary arteries are warranted.

CT coronary angiogram

CT coronary angiogram is a procedure using a multi-slice CT scanner to produce coronary artery images. Speed is extremely important in the ability to 'freeze' the heart with images. Since the heart is a rapidly moving structure, the only way to produce images of structures within the organ is for the scanning to occur as fast as or close enough to our heart beats. New generation CT machines can now perform 64, 128, 320 and even 640 slices per minute. In this procedure, intravenous dye containing iodine is used. For people with kidney disease or diabetes, kidney function may be temporarily affected. The entire CT scan can be performed when a patient holds in a single breath. The cardiac CT is more accurate than stress-testing, stress-echocardiography (ECG), or a stress-MIBI scan in determining presence of coronary blockages.

Calcium score on CT coronary scan

Calcium scoring is a technique where the extent of calcification in the coronary arteries is measured and scored. There is a direct correlation between the extent of calcium in the coronary arteries and the risk of a future cardiac event. For example, a calcium score of more than 100 is considered severe and it would be necessary to take steps to prevent further advancement of atherosclerosis and plaque formation. The higher the calcium score, the higher the likelihood of having severe stenosis (narrowing of blood vessels or valves) as well.

Nuclear scan

Nuclear scan of the heart is an imaging test that uses special cameras and a radioactive tracer to take pictures of the heart. It can detect if blood is not flowing to parts of the heart and can diagnose coronary artery disease. It can also check for damaged or dead heart muscle, possibly from a previous heart attack. Two sets of images are taken, one set at rest and another set after an exercise stress or medicine stress. Stress is used as some problems can only be detected when the heart is beating fast or working hard.

Methoxyisobutyl Isonitrile (MIBI) scan or a Cardiac Positron Emission Tomography (PET) scan are the commonly used nuclear scans. During both scans, drugs to increase heart rate or metabolism are injected followed by an injection of the radioactive tracer, before scans are performed. In the newer machines, radiation exposure is low. MIBI scan takes up to four hours to perform and the Cardiac PET can take up to half a day.

Carotid ultrasound

The carotid arteries are two large blood vessels in the neck that supply blood to the brain. Carotid artery disease screening (or carotid ultrasound) is a simple, non-invasive and painless test to measure the Carotid Intima Media Thickness. The test is performed while lying on the back. After gel is applied to the neck, a probe is used to detect images and to measure the blood flow through the carotid arteries. Doppler ultrasound technology is used to measure the amount of plaque and the speed of blood flow. It is recommended for anyone over the age of 50 years, at risk of heart disease and stroke. If carotid ultrasound is abnormal, there is a higher chance of concomitant heart disease.

Treatment Options

Medications

Commonly prescribed medications include the blood thinners and medications to control blood pressure, cholesterol and diabetes. These medications are effective only if taken long-term and consistently. The benefits are incremental, so doctors tend to combine low doses of different classes of medications if it can be tolerated. Studies have shown that progression of blockages and chances of heart attacks and strokes are much less if the right medications are used. Unfortunately, plaques or blockages cannot be reduced, thus it is better to prevent plaque build-up early than to delay treatment to a later date.

Angioplasty and stenting

Angioplasty is the medical term used to describe a procedure where arteries blocked by fatty plaque can be dilated. This is an especially important procedure as an artery that has been blocked by fat can often lead to a wide variety of heart-related conditions ranging from angina to full blown cardiac arrests.

During angioplasty, a catheter is inserted from the artery on the wrist (radial artery) or the groin (femoral artery) and used to cannulate the arteries around the heart. Once inserted, the catheter delivers the balloon to unblock the artery. Once the arteries are successfully dilated, a stent is then placed in the artery to keep the artery open. Angioplasty with stenting is a definitive treatment for artery blockage.

To put things in perspective, coronaries or heart arteries are on average only 3 mm in diameter; it takes very little plaque to impact blood or oxygen supply to the heart muscles. Thus, angioplasty and stenting are critical to opening up the delivery of oxygen to the heart muscles.

Advances in technology have resulted in more patients undergoing successful treatment with stents and avoiding open heart bypass surgery.

CABG — coronary artery bypass surgery

CABG is a surgical procedure to treat coronary artery disease. It diverts blood around narrowed or clogged parts of the major arteries to improve blood flow and oxygen supply to the heart. It is an open-heart surgery where the chest is opened. Grafts are used to divert the blood and these can be arterial grafts or venous grafts. Arterial grafts are preferred as they last longer and the standard arterial graft is the internal mammary graft from the chest wall. Graft failure is primarily due to progressive atherosclerosis over time, so repeat treatment is sometimes needed.

Complications of Ischaemic Heart Disease

Heart attack is the most serious complication of coronary artery blockage. This is because once a coronary artery is blocked, oxygen supply is interrupted and the heart muscle is destroyed. This damage may be serious and sometimes fatal. If a large portion of heart muscle is damaged, heart failure can occur. This means the heart cannot pump enough blood to meet the body's needs and will result in shortness of breath, inability to exercise, coughing at night and swelling in the legs and abdomen. Heart failure can worsen suddenly. It is important to avoid things that can trigger it. This includes excessive salt intake and missing doses of medications. Sudden arrhythmias or new heart attacks can also worsen heart failure. Thus, it is important to treat heart failure and use the appropriate medications. In very advanced heart failure, the prognosis is bleak and life expectancy is much decreased. Sudden death may occur.

Lifestyle

In general, heart health is closely linked to general health. Needless to say, the key is adequate sleep, a healthy diet and adequate exercise. Working adults while trying to survive in today's competitive environment may give up sleep and exercise and we already can see the long-term side effects of expanding waistlines and poorer health. Naturally, these lead to high blood pressure, high cholesterol and obesity, which in turn lead to higher rates of heart attack. Remember, a good night's sleep is crucial to heart health too. These are long term issues, so loss of one night of sleep will not cause chest pain the next day.

Chest pain is not a sign of a weak heart. Exercises safe for those who have weak hearts include moderate aerobic walking exercises. It is best to get the advice of your cardiologist if you already have heart problems. I have patients with weak hearts who exercise regularly and feel no worse than before, while I also have some who do not have weak hearts but don't exercise as much and can't walk very far. So, sleep well, eat healthily and exercise, above all, go for heart screening when the time comes.

The keto diet is great for weight loss but is it safe for the heart?

I have met many people who swear by the keto diet. This is a high fat, high protein and zero carb diet. While it may fight weight gain, it is definitely artery clogging and bad for the heart.

A real-life example is an athletic lady who at the age of 48 still goes for spin classes and runs half marathons. Within 3 months of starting on a keto diet, she was admitted for a heart attack. Cardiac catheterisation showed very slow flow in her heart arteries due to clogging of her micro vessels, without any blockage of the main heart arteries. Fortunately, it was a small heart attack and with cholesterol medicines and a low-fat diet, her chest pain improved. This proves that lifestyle choices have great impact on heart health.

Ways to strengthen your heart

1) Start exercising. Calculate your target heart rate and find an activity you enjoy.
2) Quit smoking. Smoking leads to heart disease and cancer. It takes 10 years after you quit for the risks to return to normal levels, so stop smoking immediately.
3) Eat healthily. Have a well-balanced diet with lean meat and fish. Fish has omega 3 which can increase good cholesterol. A low fat diet with lots of fruits and vegetables is good. Avoid processed foods.
4) Do not overeat as this leads to obesity and needless metabolic problems.
5) Moderate your stress levels to lower blood pressure and reduce your heart rate.
6) Have a good night's sleep to cap it off. Irregular sleep hours are bad for the heart and the brain.

ENDOMETRIAL AND OVARIAN CANCER

Take Home Points

1. Endometrial cancer is the most common gynaecological cancer in Singapore.
2. Any post-menopausal bleeding or abnormal vaginal bleeding in a pre-menopausal lady should be evaluated.
3. Endometrial cancer tends to present in the early stages and is mostly curable with surgery; prognosis is generally good.
4. Ovarian cancer can only be diagnosed when a biopsy is taken from the tumor and sent for laboratory assessment; there is no confirmatory scan or blood test available.
5. Ovarian cancer is usually treated by surgery with an aim to remove all organs affected by cancer, followed by chemotherapy in some cases.

Dr Pearl Tong is a Senior Consultant Obstetrician and Gynaecologist, specializing in Gynecologic Oncology, and is currently practising at the National University Hospital.

Endometrial Cancer

What is abnormal vaginal bleeding?

For ladies who have not yet reached menopause, i.e., pre-menopausal, abnormal vaginal bleeding can be defined as prolonged, heavy or frequent bleeding. Prolonged bleeding in general refers to menstrual bleeding that lasts longer than 7 days. Heavy bleeding can be subjective, if one requires pad changes more frequently than 3 hours, passes large blood clots, or experiences accidents or leakage of menstrual flow onto one's clothing despite wearing an appropriate pad. It can also be accompanied by symptoms of low blood count such as dizziness, breathlessness on exertion, tiredness objectively measured by a low hemoglobin level. Frequent bleeding refers to bleeding at intervals shorter than 21 days, or without any discernible pattern. Bleeding that occurs when one is not expected to have periods (intermenstrual bleeding) or bleeding associated with sexual intercourse (post coital bleeding) are also abnormal phenomena.

Menopause is established when one has stopped having periods for a duration longer than 12 months, from the age of 45 onwards. Upon cessation of periods, this can be associated with symptoms such as hot flushes, vaginal dryness, and mood changes. Any bleeding that occurs vaginally after menopause is abnormal and requires investigation.

What are the usual causes of post-menopausal bleeding?

There are a variety of causes for post-menopausal bleeding; it can be due to benign changes that arise from the womb lining, such as polyps in the womb lining (also known as endometrial polyps), or dryness of the womb lining/ vagina, akin to dry skin cracking and bleeding (also known as atrophy), pre-cancerous changes (such as endometrial hyperplasia) or cancerous changes (endometrial cancer). Fortunately, cancer only occurs in about 10 percent of ladies with post-menopausal bleeding. It must be noted though that the diagnosis is not based on the amount or frequency of bleeding; any post-menopausal bleeding is abnormal and ought to be investigated.

I have post-menopausal bleeding. What will the doctor do for me?

It is important to assess the entire genital tract for the cause of bleeding. The doctor will ask you some questions to determine the severity of bleeding and possible causes of this bleeding before deciding the best course of action to take. An examination is usually done in the clinic — the external genitalia is inspected, followed by inspection of the vagina walls and neck of the womb (cervix) to try to determine the source of the bleeding and to gauge the amount of bleeding. This is done by insertion of a speculum into the vagina, similar to how a PAP smear is taken. For ladies who have not had intercourse before, or are very uncomfortable about the procedure, an examination under anesthesia may be warranted.

An ultrasound of the womb and ovaries (sometimes also known as a pelvic ultrasound), may be done, to look at the womb lining, especially its thickness. A lady who had undergone menopause should have a womb lining that is thinned out, typically less than 5mm. The doctor may then decide to sample the womb lining. This can be a bedside procedure, especially for women who have delivered children before, because the neck of their wombs are usually more dilated and easily allow for the doctor to insert a thin plastic straw-like device to sample the womb lining. Otherwise, the doctor may suggest a dilatation and curettage procedure, which is done under sedation/anesthesia, usually as a day surgery case. During this procedure, the neck of the womb is dilated to allow for the womb lining to be sampled (curettage). Sometimes, a hysteroscopy may be done concurrently. This allows insertion of an instrument with a camera head to allow visualization of the womb cavity, to see if there are any causes for the bleeding, for example, polyps or tumours.

I had regular PAP smears. Why did it not pick up womb cancer?

The PAP smear test, and more recently the HPV test, are screening tests done to pick up pre cancerous conditions of the cervix, which is the neck of the womb. Womb cancer arises within the body of the womb. There are currently no screening tests recommended for the general population with regards to womb cancer. PAP smear tests, however occasionally pick up abnormal cells shed from the womb lining, prompting further investigations by your doctor.

I have been diagnosed with womb cancer!
What happens next?

This diagnosis is usually made after the womb lining has been sampled. The next step entails finding out if the cancer has spread beyond the womb, to determine the best treatment for this condition. This process is known as staging. Fortunately for womb cancer, most are discovered in the early stages and are very treatable, with a good chance of cure. Surgery is the key to staging; and is also the main treatment for womb cancer. This is usually done in conjunction with a gynaecologic oncologist — a gynaecologist who specialises in managing women with gynaecological cancer.

Surgery entails removal of the womb, fallopian tubes and ovaries, and sometimes the lymph nodes in the abdomen, to find out if the cancer has spread to those areas. This not only helps to determine the stage of the cancer, to guide further treatment but also helps to assess the risk of the cancer recurring in future. If the cancer is deemed to have higher risk of recurrence, one may be offered treatment such as radiation or chemotherapy, to try to reduce this risk.

Prior to surgery, scans are often performed in preparation for treatment planning. This may include CT (Computerised Tornography) scans of the chest, abdomen and pelvis, MRI (Magnetic Resonance Imaging) focusing on the region of the womb, or even PET (Positron Emission Tornography) CT scans that allow areas suspicious for cancer to be highlighted.

Your doctor may also mention sentinel lymph node biopsy as part of surgery. This is because in some cases, an assessment of the lymph nodes is an important factor that influences the decision for additional treatment. However, removal of lymph nodes are not without risk; these lymph nodes are near vital structures such as big blood vessels and nerves. Moreover, removal of these lymph nodes can lead to future leg swelling in some people, that can be very disturbing and lead to frequent leg infections. To cut down this risk, sentinel lymph node biopsies are performed. This procedure involves just taking one lymph node which is deemed as the "representative" of the lymph nodes in the pelvis, to determine whether the lymph nodes in the body are involved. This special lymph node is identified by injection of a special dye in the cervix after anaesthesia is administered during the surgery. Your doctor will be able to discuss with you if this procedure is applicable in your situation.

I have had surgery done for womb cancer, what happens next?

Your doctor will review the histology report (which indicates the type of cells and tissues seen and whether cancer cells are present) after the womb and other tissues sent during the surgery is analysed by the pathology lab. A stage will be assigned, and he or she will discuss with you if any further

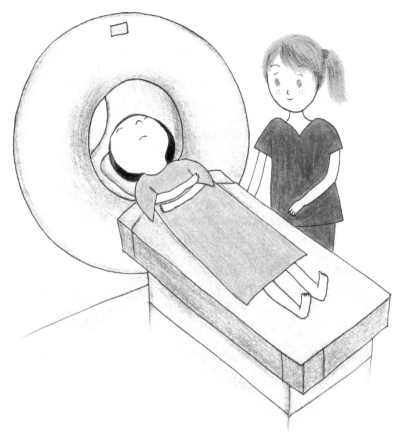

treatment such as radiation therapy or chemotherapy is required. Upon completion of treatment, be it surgery alone or with addition of other treatment, you will need to receive regular check-ups to ensure that any recurrences get picked up and treated early; and also to address any side effects of treatment.

What else do I need to be aware of after being treated for womb cancer?

A healthy lifestyle comprising of a balanced diet and regular exercise is recommended for everyone. The most common type of womb cancer is associated with obesity, high blood pressure, diabetes and high cholesterol levels. It is recommended that you adhere to the recommended yearly screening for these conditions which can be done by the general practitioner, and treated if found to be present. It has been shown in medical studies that survivors of womb cancer tend to succumb to the conditions mentioned above rather than the cancer itself.

Health supplements are usually not indicated for womb cancer survivors unless there are specific deficiencies that are identified, for example low vitamin D levels. Hormone replacement therapy can be considered for pre-menopausal patients on a case-to-case basis and this should be discussed with your treating doctors.

Sexual activity can resume usually about 2 months after surgery if the recovery process is uneventful. It is not uncommon to encounter vaginal dryness and lubricant use is advised if required.

Screening tests for cervical cancer, such as PAP smears and HPV tests are not required after a total hysterectomy as the cervix is removed during the surgery. However if you had previous pre-cancerous conditions of the cervix, it is advisable to discuss subsequent screening measures with your doctor.

Ovarian Cancer

How is it usually diagnosed?

This condition is unfortunately not easy to diagnose as its symptoms may mimic other common benign conditions. It is usually suspected when there is a lump felt in the abdomen, or when a scan done to evaluate symptoms pick up the presence of ovarian masses. There is no definitive way to determine if these lumps are benign or cancerous without getting a sample from them. Features of the lump or masses on scans, accompanying symptoms that suggest spread of these masses and blood tests such as tumour markers can help to point toward the likelihood of a lump/mass being cancer, but these are never confirmatory.

Sampling of these masses usually take place during surgery. Your doctor may discuss sending your ovarian growth for 'frozen section', which is a quick test that can be performed while you are under anaesthesia during surgery. The pathologist in the lab will do a preliminary analysis of the mass, and inform the surgeon of the nature of the mass (if the mass contains cancer cells), in order to help the surgeon decide on the next course of action. This may lead on to a staging procedure (process to determine if the cancer cells have spread to other parts of the body) if the mass was found to be cancerous. The other goal of surgery is also to remove all visible cancer tissue as part of treatment.

The staging procedure can include removal of the womb, ovary on the other side, fatty tissue attached to the intestines (known as the omentum), lymph nodes in the abdomen, appendix and biopsies of any other suspicious appearing masses in the abdomen. Alternatively, if there is no provision for frozen section or this has not been agreed upon before surgery, then another surgical procedure may be required later on for this staging process, if it is deemed to be required.

Sometimes, the cancer may appear to be widespread on the scans. Rather than doing the full cancer surgery as outlined above, your doctor may then decide to make a diagnosis first. This can be done via a minor biopsy by putting a needle through the abdomen to sample the ovarian lump, via a diagnostic keyhole surgery to assess the extent of the cancer spread and to take a biopsy to confirm that it is cancer. This can be followed by chemotherapy first, to reduce the size of the lump that is cancerous, and full cancer surgery at a later date.

What happens next after surgery?

The stage of the cancer is confirmed only after the excised specimen during surgery has been examined under the microscope by the pathologist. This then helps to determine the next best course of action. Usually, chemotherapy is required, especially in the advanced stages. A referral to the medical oncologist will then be made, for discussion and arrangement of chemotherapy.

There has also been increasing awareness that a proportion of ovarian cancer are due to specific genetic mutations. Your doctor may advise you to undergo genetic counselling and testing as this has implications on your treatment, the association of the mutation with other cancers, and the possibility of this being an inherited condition affecting your relatives.

Ovarian cancer, especially those diagnosed in Stages III and IV have a higher tendency for recurrence. This makes follow up care after completion of treatment very important. Your doctor will discuss with you the frequency of follow up, repeated scans and blood tests.

My doctor mentioned borderline ovarian tumours. What exactly are these?

Borderline ovarian tumours, as the name implies, are not cancer but they are not entirely benign. One could regard such a tumour as a growth with a tendency for recurrence and also a possibility of spread. It tends to be slower growing, can occur in younger women, and can recur many years later, compared to the usual type of ovarian cancers. It is usually managed in the same way as ovarian cancer, that is, surgery for staging and treatment purposes. However, as it tends to occur in younger women who may still desire fertility or are still far away from the average age of menopause, surgery can take a more conservative approach depending on the circumstances.

MATURE WOMANHOOD

MENOPAUSE

Take Home Points

1. Menopause happens when the usual pattern of periods stops because the ovaries no longer release eggs.
2. Although it is common to experience irregular periods during the menopausal transition period, it is important to highlight any abnormal vaginal bleeding patterns to your doctor.
3. Continue to use a safe method of birth control for pregnancy prevention in the years leading up to menopause.
4. Hormone replacement therapy is the most effective treatment for the vasomotor symptoms of menopause. Lifestyle modifications and non-hormonal treatment options may also be helpful.
5. With the right information, right lifestyle, and access to medical help, menopause can be a period of self-reflection and a chance to slow down the pace of life to focus on your health, body and mind.

The journey through a woman's lifespan brings about many seasons of change and discovery of the female body. These changes are noticeable from

Dr Lim Shu Hui is a Senior Resident in the division of Obstetrics and Gynaecology, and is currently practising at the KK Women's and Children's hospital.

Dr Celene Hui is a Consultant Obstetrician and Gynaecologist in the Minimally Invasive Surgery Unit, and is currently practising at the KK Women's and Children's hospital. She is also a Clinical Assistant Professor at Duke-NUS Medical School.

puberty, through the childbearing years, and finally during menopause — a transition that is feared by many, embraced by some, but eased into by most. Every woman's menopause journey is unique. Some may choose to go through this transition naturally, while others may seek assistance through hormone replacement therapy or other alternative treatments.

What is menopause?

Menopause happens when the usual pattern of periods stops because the ovaries no longer release eggs. This can be a natural occurrence as part of aging, or brought about by treatment such as surgical removal of the ovaries, chemotherapy or radiotherapy. Menopause is confirmed when your periods stop for at least 12 months. This happens in a majority of women between the ages of 45 to 55, with the average age being 50–51 years. Less than 1 percent of women experience menopause before the age of 40 years, and this is called premature menopause or premature ovarian insufficiency.

Fall in activity of the ovaries around menopause leads to a fall in the oestrogen levels in the body. This usually starts to occur a few months to years before the periods stop, giving rise to a period of time in a woman's life known as the menopause transition or the perimenopause.[1] During this transition period, 1 out of 2 women notice significant changes in their body. Post menopause is the time in a woman's life after menopause.

If you have undergone a hysterectomy (removal of the womb) and had your ovaries conserved, you would still undergo menopause naturally as your ovaries will stop releasing eggs. You may develop menopausal symptoms; however, it would be hard to tell when menopause is occurring as you do not have periods.

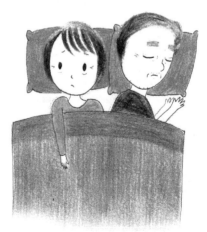

What are the common symptoms of menopause?

The most common symptoms include:

- <u>Vasomotor symptoms:</u> Vasomotor hot flushes are a sudden growing sensation of intense warmth that spreads across the whole body and face, lasting for a few minutes. The flush is sometimes concluded by profuse sweating (night sweats) that can cause a woman to wake up from her sleep or wet her clothes and bed linen. These symptoms last for approximately 4–5 years in 50 percent of women, but in 25 percent of women they may experience the symptoms for longer than 5 years.
- <u>Sleep problems:</u> Sleep problems include difficulty falling asleep at night, disrupted sleep, or waking up earlier than usual.
- <u>Mood changes:</u> Women may develop changes in their moods, such as feeling more irritable and have difficulty concentrating. Women with a past history of depression may notice their symptoms returning during the menopausal transition period.
- <u>Irregular periods:</u> In the transition to menopause, periods may become lighter, further apart and more irregular.
- <u>Vaginal dryness:</u> Due to the fall in oestrogen levels, the vagina is less lubricated and can become thin and dry. This may cause discomfort, itching or pain during sexual intercourse.
- <u>Loss of interest in having sex:</u> This may be related to vaginal dryness which causes pain and tightness during sex, or the menopausal symptoms itself which reduces the interest in having sex. It is important to note that sexual satisfaction in couples depends not only on the physical condition of each partner but also on the strength of relationship.
- <u>Joint and muscle pain:</u> The fall in oestrogen also causes more inflammation, leading to more aching and pain in the body.

Some women may experience a mild form of a few symptoms, while others experience a more severe form of many symptoms. Up to 90 percent of women will consult a doctor for advice on coping with menopausal symptoms. Every woman's experience is different and women are encouraged to seek help if these symptoms are severe enough to affect the quality of life.

How can I tell if my menstrual cycle changes are normal during the menopausal transition?

Menopausal transition is hallmarked by changes in the menstrual cycle. The early stage is marked by occasional missed periods, which later progresses to longer gaps between the periods, sometimes lasting from 60 days to 12 months. This is because ovulation, the release of eggs from the ovary, does not happen as frequently and therefore reduces the occurrence of periods until they eventually stop entirely. It can be hard to tell if your menstrual cycle changes are normal close to the menopause. In general you should consult your doctor if you have the following abnormal bleeding patterns:

- Heavy and prolonged periods
- Periods that occur more frequently than every three weeks
- Any vaginal bleeding or spotting in between menstrual cycles
- Any vaginal bleeding after sexual intercourse
- Any vaginal bleeding after the menopause, also known as post-menopausal bleeding.

These symptoms may warrant further evaluation by the gynaecologist to exclude conditions such as polyps, pre-cancer or cancer. Depending on your symptoms and risk factors, your doctor may perform a pelvic examination and order investigations such as an ultrasound scan of the pelvis, cervical smear and a biopsy of the lining of the womb.

Do I need to use birth control during the menopausal transition?

During the menopausal transition, the ovaries release eggs less frequently. The chance of pregnancy, although low, is still present. If you do not wish to get pregnant, it is advisable to continue using birth control (contraception) until menopause is confirmed with the cessation of menstruation for a duration of at least 12 months. In general, if you are above 50 years of age, it is advisable to continue using contraception for a year after your last period. However, if you are below 50 years of age when your periods stop, you are encouraged to continue using contraception for two years after your last period.

If you are on hormonal contraception, do consult your doctor on whether it is safe to continue that method during the perimenopausal period. Certain hormonal contraception options can make it difficult to determine when menopause occurs as they can affect the menstrual cycle. If you are on such forms of contraception, you may require blood tests of your hormone levels to check if you have reached menopause before stopping the contraception. Your doctor can advise you on when to stop your birth control and when to switch to safer or non-hormonal options.

How does menopause affect my bones?

The fall in oestrogen levels starting in the menopause transition period can increase susceptibility to osteoporosis, or weak bones, because the normal bone turnover cycle is impaired. This increases the risk of having fractures if there is a fall or an accident. Osteoporosis usually occurs 10–15 years after menopause, but can occur earlier if there are risk factors including inadequate calcium and vitamin D, smoking or drinking alcohol, the lack of exercise and being underweight. During the perimenopausal period, the average reduction in bone mass is about 10 percent, and continues to accelerate after menopause is established. Your risk for osteoporosis can be checked by doing bone mineral densitometry which are X-Ray scans that measure the density of your bones.

What can I do to avoid osteoporosis?

In order to avoid bone weakness, you are advised to take enough calcium by taking calcium tablets or milk, and ensure that you get enough vitamin D by exposing yourself to sunlight or taking vitamin D tablets. It is also important to stay active and do weight bearing exercises to strengthen your bones and muscles, such as dancing, tai chi, skipping, jogging, stair climbing. Smoking and drinking should also be discontinued as these can reduce your bone density.

What are the treatment options available for osteoporosis?

If you are diagnosed with osteoporosis, your doctor may calculate your risk for having fractures. If you have other menopausal symptoms, you may also be offered hormone replacement therapy as this has been proven to improve bone mineral density and help to treat the other troublesome symptoms of menopause. Other treatments that can be discussed with you include specific treatments for osteoporosis such as bisphosphonates, selected oestrogen receptor modulators, recombinant human parathyroid hormone, denosumab — all of which are effective options for osteoporosis.

What is my risk of heart disease after menopause?

Cardiovascular disease is the disease of the heart and blood vessels. The risk of developing cardiovascular disease increases when oestrogen levels decline, and it is the most common cause of death in both women and men. Risk factors for cardiovascular disease include: a family history of cardiovascular disease, high blood pressure, smoking, diabetes, abnormal cholesterol levels and obesity. Men under the age of 40 have twice the risk of developing cardiovascular disease compared to women, however this advantage in women is gradually lost with increasing age. Adjustment of lifestyle by maintaining a healthy diet and exercising, while controlling any long-term medical problems, are essential in decreasing your cardiovascular risk. If you experience premature menopause, you may be offered hormone replacement therapy until the average age of menopause (50 years) to reduce the risk of cardiovascular disease.

Will my urinary incontinence worsen after menopause?

Urinary incontinence is the inability to control your urine. Although urinary incontinence is not a major symptom of the menopause and perimenopausal transition, it can worsen in some women with increasing age. Urinary incontinence occurs because of laxity of your pelvic muscles leading to stress incontinence (leaking of urine when you cough, laugh or sneeze) and is more common in women who have had vaginal deliveries. You may also experience urge incontinence (leaking of urine before you make it to the toilet, associated with urgency) which is caused by an overactive bladder. Women may also find they experience a mix of both stress and urge incontinence. If this is a bothersome symptom, you should visit your doctor for further evaluation and treatment. Kegel's exercises to strengthen the pelvic floor and vaginal oestrogen creams may help to relieve these symptoms. However if these are ineffective, you may be advised to start medications or undergo surgery to reinforce the pelvic floor.

How can I stay healthy after menopause?

The transition to menopause and knowledge of its associated risks brings to light the importance of taking care of our bodies. Some lifestyle changes to follow as you ease into this phase of life include:

Association of Women
Doctors (Singapore)

- Quitting smoking and drinking
- Eating a healthy and balanced diet — high in fibre, fruits, vegetables, wholegrains, low in fats, cholesterol and refined carbohydrates
- Ensuring that you have enough calcium and vitamin D
- Maintaining your weight within the healthy BMI range (18.5–24.9)
- Doing weight-bearing exercises at least 3 times a week
- Keeping a healthy social life, or finding a meaningful hobby to keep yourself occupied
- Taking part in mentally stimulating activities such as reading or doing crossword puzzles to ensure that your mind stays active
- Wearing loose clothes at night, and sleeping in a well-ventilated room that is sufficiently cool to reduce night sweats
- Avoiding triggers for hot flushes such as caffeine, spicy food and alcohol
- Getting enough rest, reducing stress levels to avoid mood swings
- Participating in the national screening programme for breast cancer, cervical cancer and colorectal cancer.

What is hormone replacement therapy (HRT)?

Hormone replacement therapy (HRT) may be prescribed for the treatment of symptoms related to menopause. Most of the symptoms are caused by the withdrawal of oestrogen from the body, hence hormone replacement therapy targets the root cause of these symptoms. HRT is usually given as a combination of estrogen and progesterone, or estrogen alone if your womb has been removed. The hormones can be given in the form of tablets, gels, patches, pessaries, or intrauterine devices. Depending on your medical history, your symptoms and needs, your doctor will choose a treatment option that is best and safest for you.

What are the risks and benefits of HRT?

HRT is a highly effective treatment for troublesome menopausal symptoms, such as hot flushes, night sweats and vaginal dryness. It is also helpful in preventing osteoporosis. It can also reduce the risk of cardiovascular disease, although it should not be prescribed solely for this purpose. The effect of HRT on dementia and muscle mass is unknown. Common side effects of HRT include headache, breast tenderness, abdominal bloating and muscle cramps. There are also health risks that come with the use of HRT, but the absolute risks are small. For conditions such as breast cancer and stroke, the risks are typically smaller than the risks associated with obesity and smoking.

The risk of breast cancer may be increased when taking an oestrogen and progesterone formulation. However, careful selection of the type and form of hormone used can mitigate this risk. The increase in risk of breast cancer is related to the duration of HRT, and this risk is reduced when HRT is discontinued. Your doctor would therefore advise you to use the lowest effective dose of HRT to help you cope with your menopausal symptoms for the shortest duration of time.

When HRT is taken in the tablet form, it also increases your risk of forming blood clots in the legs by 2–3 times. These blood clots are dangerous as they can potentially travel to the lungs or brain, causing fatal consequences. It can increase the risk of stroke, though the absolute risk of stroke is low if you are young (below the age of 60). These risks may be minimised by taking HRT in the patch or gel form, maintaining a healthy BMI, and avoiding smoking and drinking.

What kind of HRT is suitable for me?

HRT formulations are individualised depending on your symptoms, age and risk factors. If you have a womb, you will be prescribed a combination of oestrogen and progestogen (combined HRT). This is because if oestrogen is given alone, it causes thickening of the womb lining, which may lead to bleeding or promote the growth of precancerous cells within the lining. This is known as endometrial hyperplasia. Progesterone opposes this action, and is thus prescribed alongside oestrogen to protect the womb lining. This can be prescribed as a tablet form, patches or an intrauterine device.

If HRT is started before established menopause or within 12 months of your last period, then it is given in a cyclical fashion — 21 tablets every 28 days, which leads to regular monthly bleeding similar to if you were to take contraceptive pills. If HRT is started after established menopause (more than 12 months from the last period), a continuous formulation may be prescribed with no pill-free interval and hence no withdrawal bleeding. Tibolone is a prescription medication given continuously to women who are >12 months from their last period. It is similar to taking combined HRT.

On initiation of HRT, there may be irregular vaginal bleeding within the first 3 months which is expected to resolve spontaneously. If the abnormal bleeding persists beyond 3 months, medical consultation should be sought. If you have had a hysterectomy (womb removal), then oestrogen-only HRT will be given as progesterone is not required to protect the womb lining, and there are less risks. While on HRT, there will be regular appointments with your doctor to assess the effectiveness and tolerability of the medications and to review for any adverse events. The treatments may be adapted based on your changing symptoms.

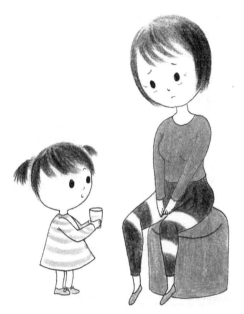

What non-hormonal treatment options are available for menopausal symptoms?

It is important to note that the first-line management of menopausal symptoms still entails simple lifestyle changes (see section on "How can I stay healthy after menopause?"). If these fail, hormone replacement therapy is the most effective treatment for menopausal symptoms. However, there are also non-hormonal medical treatments and psychological treatments that may be considered if you are not keen on taking HRT, or if you are not suitable for HRT.[2]

Herbal preparations

Herbal preparations such as isoflavones or black cohosh are thought to be effective in relieving vasomotor symptoms like hot flushes, but there are many preparations on the market, there is uncertainty about their safety, and they may interact with other medications. St John's wort may also be effective, however there is currently insufficient evidence on the appropriate dosage and concentration, and there are potential serious interactions with other long-term medications. Although these treatments are marketed as 'herbal', or 'natural', this does not necessarily mean they are safe and they may sometimes cause some unpleasant side effects. It is recommended that you consult your doctor for more information before commencing on any of these treatments.

Psychological treatments

Psychological treatments such as cognitive behavioural therapy (CBT) have been shown to be effective in treating the low mood or anxiety that arise from menopause. It has also been shown to reduce the impact of hot flushes and night sweats.[3] This is a type of treatment that focuses on identifying underlying negative thoughts and replacing them with more objective, realistic thoughts.

Prescription medication

Prescription medication that are used for other conditions have been effective when used to treat certain symptoms of menopause.

Gabapentin or pregabalin, used to treat epilepsy, neurogenic pain and migraine, can reduce hot flushes and improve quality of sleep associated with menopause. Clonidine is a treatment for high blood pressure, which can be used to reduce hot flushes and night sweats. As it is not a hormonal preparation, it does not affect hormone levels and hence does not increase risk of breast cancer. There is insufficient evidence that anti-depressant medications such as SSRI (selective serotonin reuptake inhibitors) and SNRI (serotonin and norepinephrine reuptake inhibitors) should be given in psychological conditions related to menopause. These medications may have some effectiveness for hot flushes, but are not licensed for this use. SSRIs such as paroxetine and fluoxetine should not be offered to women with breast cancer who are taking tamoxifen as this reduces the effectiveness of tamoxifen.

What are the options available for vaginal dryness?

Vaginal moisturisers and lubricants can reduce vaginal dryness and are available without a prescription. Water-based lubricants are recommended when used together with condoms as oil-based lubricants can damage the latex and reduce the efficacy of condoms in preventing pregnancy as well as sexually transmitted infections. Vaginal moisturisers allow vaginal tissue to retain moisture. Hand and body lotions are not recommended as vaginal moisturisers and can cause vaginal irritation.

If these are ineffective, you may consider the use of topical vaginal oestrogen therapy. Vaginal oestrogen therapy often comes in either a cream or tablet form. Vaginal oestrogen therapy is highly effective in treating vaginal dryness and effects are seen within a few weeks of initiating treatment. Only a very small amount of oestrogen is absorbed into the body and hence, the risk of side effects is much lower.

References

1. Delamater L and Santoro N. Management of the perimenopause. *Clin Obstet Gynecol* 2018; 61(3): 419–432. doi:10.1097/GRF.0000000000000389.
2. El Khoudary S, Aggarwal B, Beckie T *et al.* Menopause transition and cardiovascular disease risk: implications for timing of early prevention: a scientific statement from the American Heart Association. *Circulation* 2020; 142(25). doi:10.1161/cir.0000000000000912.
3. Norton S, Chilcot J and Hunter, M. Cognitive-behavior therapy for menopausal symptoms (hot flushes and night sweats). *Menopause* 2014; 21(6): 574–578. doi: 10.1097/gme.0000000000000095.

Further Reading

Hormone Replacement Therapy (HRT): Alternatives. National Health Service, UK; 2019 Sep 9. Available at: https://www.nhs.uk/conditions/hormone-replacement-therapy-hrt/alternatives/.

Ji MX and Yu Q. Primary osteoporosis in postmenopausal women. *Chronic Dis Transl Med* 2015; 1(1): 9–13. doi:10.1016/j.cdtm.2015.02.006.

Menopause: diagnosis and management, NICE Guidelines NG23. National Institute for Health and Care Excellence; 2015 Nov 12. Available at: https://www.nice.org.uk/guidance/ng23.

Norton S, Chilcot J and Hunter, M. Cognitive-behavior therapy for menopausal symptoms (hot flushes and night sweats). *Menopause* 2014; 21(6): 574–578. doi: 10.1097/gme.0000000000000095.

Taylor HS, Pal L and Seli E. *Speroff's Clinical Gynecologic Endocrinology and Infertility* (Ninth Edition). Netherlands: Wolters Kluwer (2020).

DEMENTIA

Take Home Points

1. Dementia is a pathological process and is different from normal aging.
2. Short term memory loss is only 1 out of 6 domains which can be affected by a dementing process.
3. Behavioural and psychological symptoms of dementia are common and include: low interest in activities, depression, agitation and delusions. These behaviours can be distressing to both patient and family members caring for them.
4. Nonpharmacological management for dementia includes a good support system, cognitive rehabilitation, social engagement and maintenance of physical function.
5. Pharmacological management of dementia can potentially reduce the severity of cognitive decline and compress the number of years in which the patient will spend in severe stages where increased assistance is required.

Dr Sri Karpageshwary is a Senior Resident in the division of Geriatric Medicine in Singhealth.

Dementia is a neurodegenerative disorder of the brain with increased incidence seen with advancing age. Dementia is a heterogenous disease process due to multiple factors such as age, an individual's pre-existing medical conditions and cognitive reserve. Classically, dementia is associated with memory impairment, particularly with respect to short term memory loss.

However, dementia can affect multiple domains, resulting in functional impairment and hence affecting one's ability of self-care and presence in the community. These include impairment in complex attention, executive function, perceptual motor tasks, language and social cognition.

Patients with dementia display difficulty completing routine tasks which they used to be able to do with ease, struggle with navigating familiar routes and may get lost easily; these also lead them to display increased anxiety. They may also display lapses in judgment and have poor decision making in which their loved one is able to observe a clear intra individual change from their baseline.

What are the risk factors for developing dementia? I am generally a healthy person.

Age is the greatest risk factor for dementia with incidence increasing exponentially after 65 years old.

Medical conditions that serve as risk factors include hypertension and diabetes; these conditions stimulate a chronic inflammatory state within the body hence having harmful effect on cognitive function.

Vices such as smoking and physical inactivity is also implicated with dementia. Smoking is known to contain neurotoxins and predisposes one to strokes and other diseases.

Exercise is well backed by research as being a protective factor, with observational studies highlighting the inverse relationship between exercise and the risk of dementia. In addition, exercise has multitude of benefits in the elderly, including improving balance, reducing falls and improving one's mood. Hence adopting a healthy lifestyle and controlling pre-existing medical conditions is key to preventing and delaying the onset of dementia.

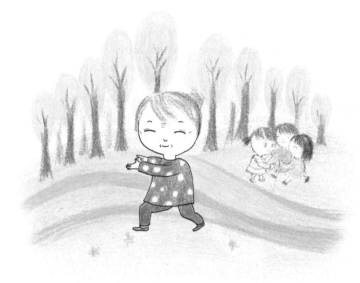

My dad has been diagnosed with dementia, are there any medications which can help him? I have heard that it is not a curable disease.

There is no curative agent for dementia management. The current FDA approved medications target biochemical abnormalities in the brain but do not serve to modify the underlying neuropathology and subsequent progression. In this same vein, there is no medication to reverse the cognitive deficits displayed by patients with dementia. Medications can slow down the deterioration process of dementia. However, this varies with individuals as it depends on how the patient responds to the drug.

Dementia care is best defined as one that is patient centred where a needs assessment is carried out by the attending geriatrician. Interventions are tailored within the domains of medical, cognitive, emotional and psychosocial. The risk that arises due to decreased safety awareness are also assessed and promptly addressed during clinical visit including that of malnutrition and home safety.

Hence the goal will be to maximise function and cognition utilising both nonpharmacological and pharmacological intervention. Non pharmacological interventions include social engagement, cognitive stimulation via cognitive exercises and rehabilitation, as well as physical activity tailored to the patient.

The aim is then to improve everyday functioning of the patient by setting specific goals and devising strategies to attain them done in a multi disciplinary fashion. Pharmacological interventions include cognitive enhancers which serve to modulate neurotransmitters in the brain as well as optimisation of cardiovascular risk factors such as diabetes and hypertension.

I have heard that patients with dementia can have strange behaviours, is that accurate?

It is common for patients with dementia to exhibit behavioural symptoms which is termed as Behavioural and Psychological symptoms of Dementia (BPSD).

The presence of these symptoms can be more prevalent as the dementia progresses. However in certain dementia types such as frontotemporal dementia, behavioural symptoms serve to be a prominent feature early in the disease course. Common symptoms which are persistent include depression and apathy while psychotic symptoms of hallucinations and features of hyperactivity displayed as agitation serve to be most distressing. Certain types of dementia have an affinity towards behavioural patterns such as Lewy body dementia which is associated with vivid visual hallucinations and frontotemporal dementia which is associated with disinhibition.

Wow that sounds challenging! How do we support our loved one if they develop BPSD?

BPSD symptoms are not just challenging for the patients but are equally or more burdensome for the caregivers. It is associated with increased risk of institutionalisation and death.

Firstly, the physician will evaluate for the presence of reversible causes of behavioural change, including visual and hearing loss as well as inappropriate sensory stimulation which may be distressing to the patient.

After the above is addressed, the persisting BPSD symptoms are individually assessed to formulate a patient centred plan which is regularly evaluated during follow-up.

Medications are administered when symptoms cause excessive distress to the patient and family, placing the patient at an increased risk of an undesirable outcome. Prior to initiation, the risk benefit profile including side effects should be explained and close monitoring done at follow-up visits.

It is important to be cognisant that symptoms are beyond the control of the individual and the expression is secondary to the underlying dementing process. Hence establishing a good support system with adequate understanding of the disease process is paramount.

Since my dad has been diagnosed with dementia, does that mean I am at risk? Is there any way I can get tested?

Genetic testing is not recommended for families of patients with dementia. Although certain genes have been associated with dementia such as in Alzheimer dementia and frontotemporal dementia, the clinical implications are not sufficiently clear for routine testing to be implemented.

COMMON EYE CONDITIONS

Take Home Points

1. Refractive errors and dry eye disease are the most common and underdiagnosed eye conditions.
2. The type and frequency of eye conditions may differ with age, ethnicity and gender.
3. Myopia can be prevented or its progression can be slowed down, by practising good eye habits from young. While there is no prevention for many other eye conditions such as age-related macular degeneration or cataracts, lifestyle modifications can reduce the risk or slow down the progression of the condition.
4. Appropriate eye screening is advised for conditions with genetic basis and family history, such as glaucoma, which may be asymptomatic in the early stages.
5. Seek professional eye consult early if you have persistent or worsening eye symptoms.

Dr Annabel Chew is a Senior Consultant Ophthalmologist, specializing in Glaucoma, and is currently practising at the Singapore National Eye Centre. She is also a Clinical Assistant Professor at Duke-NUS Medical School.

Dr Yap Zhu Li is a Consultant Ophthalmologist, specializing in Glaucoma and Complex Cataract Surgery, and is currently practising at the Singapore National Eye Centre. She is also a Clinical Assistant Professor at Duke-NUS Medical School.

Dry Eye Disease

What is dry eye disease (DED)?

Dry eye disease (DED) is a multifactorial disease in which the tear film is abnormal. Our tears are composed of 3 layers — water, an outer oily layer, and an inner mucus layer. DED occurs when the eye does not produce sufficient tears, or when the tear composition is abnormal, or when tears evaporate too quickly.

What causes DED?

It is a multifactorial disease. Some causative factors include:

- Ageing — tear production tends to decrease with age
- Hormonal changes due to pregnancy or menopause
- Problem with the oil glands along the eyelid margins (meibomian gland dysfunction) resulting in blockage of the oil glands or excessive oil production
- Eyelid conditions such as entropion (when the eyelids are turned in), or ectropion (when the eyelids are turned out)
- Blinking less in conditions such as Parkinson's disease, stroke or Bell's palsy
- Medical conditions resulting in inflammation or damage to the lacrimal gland (which produces the water component of the tears) or conjunctiva (tissue that covers the surface of the eye) such as Sjogren's syndrome, rheumatoid arthritis, systemic lupus erythematosis, graft versus host disease, thyroid disorders etc.
- Medications such as antihistamines, nasal decongestants, birth control pills, antidepressants, Parkinson's medications
- Preservatives in topical eyedrops
- Contact lens use
- History of refractive surgery.

What are the symptoms of DED?

Symptoms of DED include:

- Eye redness and irritation
- Burning sensation in your eye

- Stringy mucus in your eye
- Transient blurred vision
- Tearing due to reflex tearing.

How is DED diagnosed?

Your ophthalmologist can diagnose DED by taking a detailed history and performing an eye examination. The following assessments may be performed:

- Checking the ocular surface for damage with stains
- Checking the tear film stability by measuring the tear film break up time
- Checking the eyelid structure and blink mechanism
- Schirmer's test to measure the tear production.

What are the complications of DED?

Most people with mild DED have no long-term problems. Severe untreated DED can lead to eye infection, corneal ulcer, and damage to the surface of the eyes, which may result in visual loss.

How is DED managed?

Lifestyle modifications:

- Increase dietary omega-3 fatty acid intake. This is found in oily fish (such as salmon, sardine, tuna etc), and in flaxseeds
- Avoid smoking
- Avoid dry atmosphere and use a humidifier in the room
- Blink more frequently; take frequent breaks from screen time.

Treatment options:

- Regular use of lubricating eye drops or ointments
- Warm compress and cleaning your eyelids with eyelid cleansers or diluted baby shampoo for meibomian gland dysfunction
- Topical anti-inflammatory drops for severe dry eyes
- Punctal plugs to block off the tear ducts

- Eyelid surgery for eyelid problems
- Managing the underlying medical condition.

Cataract

What is cataract?

Cataract is the clouding of your eye's natural lens which reduces visual clarity as it worsens.

What are the symptoms of cataract?

Gradual (usually over months to years), painless, progressive constant blurry vision is the most common symptom of cataract. Other symptoms include glare, poor night vision, faded colours (brownish or yellow tint), double vision and frequent changing of glasses.

Am I at risk of getting cataract?

The vast majority of cataracts are age-related, so everyone eventually develops cataracts, similar to white hair or wrinkles! There are other associated conditions which may cause it to occur earlier in life. These conditions include diabetes, chronic steroid use, high myopia, eye trauma or cigarette smoking.

Can I prevent the condition and if so, how?

Cataract development is part of the aging process and cannot be completely prevented. The development can however be slowed down by modifying some habits. These include: wearing sunglasses to reduce UV exposure, avoiding steroid eyedrops unless specifically prescribed by an ophthalmologist, living a healthy lifestyle and controlling any health issues that may speed up cataract development (such as diabetes).

How do I manage the condition?

Management options vary according to how advanced the cataract is and if the person's activities of daily living are affected. There are currently no medications to 'cure' or slow down cataract formation. In some cases, changing your glasses may help for a period of time. Cataract surgery with intraocular lens implant is the definitive treatment for cataracts.

How is cataract surgery performed?

The main technique used to remove cataract is phacoemulsification. It is performed by making microscopic incisions in the periphery of the cornea (the transparent front surface of the eye) and introducing an ultrasonic device through this opening into the eye. This device uses ultrasound power to break the cloudy lens up into small pieces and this facilitates removal from the eye. Cataract is always removed via this ultrasound device and not by a laser, though in some cases, laser may be used for parts of the surgery.

After the cataract is entirely removed, an artificial lens implant is inserted into the same position. This method of cataract surgery takes an average 15 to 30 minutes. In more difficult cases, it could take more than 30 minutes. Anaesthetic eyedrops and sometimes an injection will be given to keep pain to a minimum.

What are the different options for intraocular lens?

Monofocal and multifocal artificial lens implants are available. Your ophthalmologist will discuss with you and recommend the type of implant that is most suitable for you.

Standard monofocal lenses:

- Most commonly implanted lenses, with equal power in all regions of the lens
- Provide good overall vision at a specific distance (mainly for distant vision)
- Reading glasses will be required
- Suitable for people who are comfortable wearing reading glasses.

Multifocal lenses:

- Provide good distance and near vision without glasses
- Convenient as both near and intermediate vision (for fixed distances) can be clearer using these lenses

- However, some people may find it difficult to read fine print, especially in dim light, and may experience glare and haloes which may be bothersome
- This lens should be used in both eyes
- Suitable for people who want to reduce their dependence on glasses for far and near vision.

How do I look after my eye after Cataract surgery?

After the operation, you will need to:

- Clean the skin around the eye for the first week after surgery with sterile water and cotton balls
- Keep your eye covered with an eye shield on the day of surgery and while sleeping for one week
- Prevent contaminated water from entering the eye
- Instil the post-operative eyedrops as prescribed
- Do not rub your eye.

Will cataract recur after surgery?

No. Cataract surgery removes the original cataractous lens and it will never recur. However, vision can deteriorate after cataract surgery for a variety of other reasons. Most commonly, 20–30 percent of patients experience some decline in their vision in the years after surgery due to the bag holding the implanted lens becoming cloudy. A simple laser procedure can be done to remove the cloudy bag. Other causes of vision deterioration after cataract surgery include the development of other eye conditions such as glaucoma, age-related macular degeneration etc. If you do experience vision deterioration, do not hesitate to see an ophthalmologist for further assessment.

Refractive Errors

What are refractive errors?

Refractive errors are a type of vision problem that makes it hard to see clearly. They happen when the shape of your eye keeps light from focusing correctly on your retina (a light-sensitive layer of tissue in the back of your eye). There are different types of refractive errors, namely:

- Myopia or short-sightedness, where far-away objects look blurry (very common in Singapore with >80% of the young adult population having the condition)
- Hyperopia or long-sightedness, where nearby objects look blurry
- Astigmatism where both far and near objects look blurry. It can be due to an irregular eye surface (cornea) or lens.

Am I at risk of getting refractive errors?

Myopia is caused by a combination of genetic and environmental factors. A family history of myopia predisposes one to it. Other habits such as long periods of detailed or close work and childhood illnesses may also influence the progression of myopia. Long duration of near work such as reading, studying and computer usage also increase the risk of myopia. The risk of myopia is higher in children and usually decreases as one gets older though there are people who have myopia progression in their 20s and 30s. In older people who have increasing myopia, cataract is often the culprit.

Hyperopia is usually present at birth and tends to be genetic.

Astigmatism often occurs with myopia and hyperopia. It is often genetic but may develop later in life due to trauma, injury, excessive eye rubbing or after eye surgery.

Can I prevent refractive errors and if so, how?

Myopia cannot be reversed or cured, but it can be slowed down or prevented. Near work is unavoidable, so practising healthy eye habits is essential. Take frequent breaks to rest your eyes and spend more times outdoors. This is especially crucial in children so parents should start their children young and encourage them to practise good eye habits to prevent myopia from occurring or worsening.

Hyperopia is often present from birth and cannot be prevented. It is easily corrected with eyeglasses or contact lenses and some even consider surgery.

How do I manage the condition?

Refractive errors are the most common type of vision problem and easily corrected with the use of eyeglasses or contact lenses, which is why timely eye examinations are so important.

Presbyopia

What is presbyopia?

Presbyopia is the gradual loss of the eyes' ability to focus on nearby objects.

Am I at risk of getting presbyopia?

Presbyopia becomes noticeable by the early 40s and continues to worsen until around the age of 65. People often notice it when they have to adjust the distance at which they hold their phones and books when reading as they have blurred vision at their normal reading distance and experience eye strain or even headaches after reading or doing close-up work.

Can I prevent the condition and if so, how?

Unfortunately, it is part of the natural process of aging. Being farsighted or having certain diseases such as diabetes, multiple sclerosis or cardiovascular risk can increase one's risk of premature presbyopia. Certain drugs are also associated with premature presbyopia such as antidepressants, antihistamines and diuretics.

How do I manage the condition?

A basic eye examination by an ophthalmologist can confirm presbyopia and the condition can be corrected with spectacles or contact lenses and in some cases, surgery.

Glaucoma

What is glaucoma?

Glaucoma is a disease that causes damage to the optic nerve (eye nerve), that is often associated with raised eye pressure.

It is a leading cause of irreversible blindness worldwide. As the population ages with increased life expectancy, the number of people with glaucoma worldwide is estimated to increase to 111.8 million in 2040.

Most forms of glaucoma have no symptoms in the early stages, and they often remain undetected until they progress to a more advanced stage with extensive vision loss, hence glaucoma is known as the 'silent thief of sight'.

Glaucoma tends to affect both eyes, sometimes one eye more than the other. Glaucoma cannot be cured, but if it is detected and treated early, vision loss may be slowed down and blindness may be prevented.

What causes glaucoma?

Aqueous humour is a fluid which provides nutrients to the eye and maintains its shape. There is a delicate balance between the production and drainage of this fluid and glaucoma is usually caused by a build-up of this fluid within the eye. This can happen when the drainage system is not functioning properly, or when there is too much fluid being produced, resulting in raised eye pressure, and subsequent damage to the optic nerve. The optic nerve is responsible for sending visual impulses from the eye to the brain.

What are the types of glaucoma?

Glaucoma can be classified into primary or secondary disease. Primary glaucoma is not associated with other diseases, whereas secondary glaucoma is a result of other diseases (arising from uncontrolled diabetes, or following an eye injury, or chronic steroid use etc).

It can also be classified into open angle or angle closure disease. Primary open angle glaucoma is the most common form of glaucoma. The drainage angles are open, however the drainage system is impaired, resulting in raised eye pressure. In angle closure glaucoma, the drainage angles are narrow or closed, preventing the fluid from reaching the drainage system, again resulting in raised eye pressure.

It is rare but possible for babies and children to have glaucoma. It can occur at birth, or develop later on in life. This can be a result of a defect in the development of the eye, or other eye diseases (such as a tumour, or following an eye injury, infection etc).

What are the symptoms of glaucoma?

Most forms of the glaucoma are chronic and develop gradually. Symptoms of chronic glaucoma include:

- No symptoms in the early stages
- Loss of peripheral vision or tunnel vision

- Blurred vision
- Blindness in end-stage glaucoma.

Acute glaucoma is rarer and occurs when there is a sudden rise in the eye pressure. Symptoms of acute glaucoma include:

- Eye pain and redness
- Severe headache
- Nausea and vomiting
- Seeing halos around lights.

Symptoms of childhood glaucoma that develop within the first few years include:

- Enlarged eyes
- Cornea cloudiness
- Tearing
- Light sensitivity.

What are the risk factors of glaucoma?

Risk factors for glaucoma include:

- Older age (over 40 years old)
- High eye pressure
- Family history of glaucoma
- Male gender for primary open angle glaucoma, female gender for primary angle closure glaucoma
- African, East Asian, and Inuit ethnicity
- Myopia (short-sightedness) or hyperopia (long-sightedness)
- Hypertension, Diabetes Mellitus
- Long-term steroid use
- Eye injury
- Obstructive sleep apnoea
- Migraine.

Can glaucoma be prevented?

Glaucoma cannot be prevented. However early detection with regular eye checks will allow for timely treatment to preserve the remaining vision.

- You should have regular eye examination if you have a family history of glaucoma, or if you have other risk factors for glaucoma.
- You should go for a baseline eye check if you are over 40 years old.

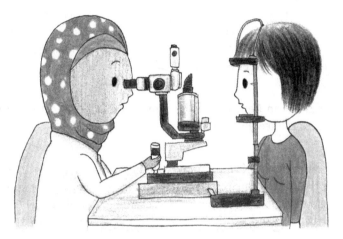

How is glaucoma diagnosed?

Your ophthalmologist can diagnose glaucoma by performing an eye examination, and assessing the following:

- Tonometry to measure your eye pressure
- Gonioscopy to check your drainage angles
- Optic nerve examination
- Visual field test
- Optical coherence tomography scan of the optic nerve.

How is glaucoma managed?

Glaucoma is a chronic condition that requires life-long review. It cannot be cured. Once the optic nerve is damaged, the damage is permanent and vision loss is irreversible. The aim of treatment is to lower the eye pressure to a safe level, to preserve the remaining vision.

Treatment options include:

Medications
There are different forms of medications used in glaucoma treatment. They reduce the eye pressure by reducing the fluid production in the eye, or increasing the fluid drainage. Eyedrops are most commonly used, and can be used long-term. Oral medications or intravenous injections are usually only used for a short period of time to quickly lower the eye pressure.

Laser
Laser operation can be used to open up the angles, or increase the fluid drainage, or to reduce the fluid production in the eye.

Surgery
There are different surgical options including creating an alternative route for fluid in the eye to drain out (trabeculectomy or tube implant surgery), or implanting a device into the angle to increase the fluid drainage (minimally invasive glaucoma surgery).

Depending on the type of glaucoma you have, your ophthalmologist will advise which treatment option is the best for you.

How do I instil my glaucoma eyedrops?

It is important to use your glaucoma eye drops every day in the prescribed frequency, even on the day of your eye check. If you need to instil more than 1 type of medication, please wait at least 5 minutes between instilling the different drops. Do place your finger against the lower eyelid where it meets your nose (punctum occlusion) for at least 3 minutes following eyedrop instillation to maximize the absorption into the eye and reduce the absorption into the bloodstream. Do get a new prescription in advance before your eyedrops run out. If you encounter any problems with your eyedrops, please consult your ophthalmologist urgently before stopping your eyedrops.

Age-related Macular Degeneration

What is age-related macular degeneration (AMD)?

Age-related macular degeneration (AMD) is a chronic medical condition that develops as the eye ages, where there is damage to the macula (centre part of the retina). It is a leading cause of irreversible blindness worldwide in people 50 years or older. The macula is responsible for clear central vision, and allows us to see details clearly. In AMD, there is loss of central vision, and the peripheral side vision is usually not affected. AMD can affect one or both eyes.

What are the types of AMD?

There are 2 types of AMD: dry and wet.

Dry AMD is more common, and affects around 90 percent of people with AMD. In dry AMD, the macula forms yellow deposits (drusens), and slowly gets thinner and more damaged with age.

Wet AMD is less common. In wet AMD, abnormal blood vessels grow under the retina and can bleed or leak fluid, resulting in damage to the macula. Vision loss can occur suddenly in wet AMD.

What are the symptoms of AMD?

Symptoms of AMD include:

- Distorted vision (straight lines appear wavy)
- Gradual or sudden onset of loss of central vision
- Blind spots in central vision.

What are the risk factors of AMD?

Risk factors for AMD include:

- Increased age
- Smoking
- Obesity
- Cardiovascular disease
- Family history of AMD.

Can AMD be prevented?

AMD cannot be prevented. However, you can reduce your risk of getting the disease by not smoking, eating a healthy balanced diet with fruits and vegetables, and protecting your eyes from ultraviolet light with protective sunglasses. Also, early detection through regular eye checks will allow for timely treatment.

How is AMD diagnosed?

Your ophthalmologist can diagnose AMD by performing an eye examination, and assessing the following:

- Dilated examination of the retina and macula
- Optical coherence tomography scan of the macula
- Angiography of the retina to detect abnormal blood vessels. A fluorescent dye is injected into a vein, and photographs of the eye are taken as the dye passes through the retina blood vessels.

How do I test my vision with the Amsler Grid?

The Amsler Grid is a chart that consists of many squares. If you have AMD, you can use the Amsler Grid to monitor your vision every day. Wear your reading glasses, and hold the chart in front of you at a reading distance. Cover one eye, so that you are testing one eye at a time. Focus your eye on the centre dot, and look at the surrounding lines. If the lines appear wavy or distorted or blurred, or if you see a black patch, please see your ophthalmologist for an eye check.

How is AMD treated?

There is no treatment for dry AMD. In some forms of dry AMD, progression of the disease may be slowed down with a high-dose vitamin and mineral supplements (AREDS2 supplements) that contain lutein, vitamin C, vitamin E, zinc, copper, and zeaxanthin. Supplements containing beta-carotene should not be taken by smokers or former smokers as there is an increased risk of lung cancer.

Wet AMD may lead to irreversible visual loss. Treatment options include:

Injection of medications into the eye
The medications used are called anti-vascular endothelial growth factor (anti-VEGF) medications. They help to stop the growth of the abnormal blood vessels, and may help to stabilize the vision. Repeated injections are

usually required. While most people's vision can be maintained with anti-VEGF treatment, only one third will have visual improvement. Some people may not respond to the treatment at all.

Laser
Laser is used to destroy the abnormal blood vessels.

Your ophthalmologist will advise which treatment option is the best for you.

Further Reading

Buckley RJ. Assessment and management of dry eye disease. *Eye* (Lond) 2018 Feb; 32(2): 200–203.

Tham YC, Li X, Wong TY *et al.* Global prevalence of glaucoma and projections of glaucoma burden through 2040 — a systematic review and meta-analysis. *Ophthalmology* 2014; 121: 2081–2090.

THE PSYCHOLOGICAL IMPACT OF AGEING

Do not go gentle into that good night.
Rage, rage against the dying of the light.
— Dylan Thomas

Take Home Points

1. Ageing is a natural, physical process, with a definitive impact on our mental well-being and lifestyle.
2. Understanding the psychological and emotional impact of ageing is important to help us maintain a positive attitude in our golden years.
3. Barriers to achieving this may include unhealthy coping strategies.
4. Methods of safeguarding mental and physical well-being is important to maintaining a healthy state of mind during such times.
5. Practical end-of-life matters should also be discussed in an open manner with those you trust.

Dr Tina Tan is a Consultant Psychiatrist, specializing in Geriatric Psychiatry, and is currently practising at the Better Life Clinic.

What is Ageing?

Simply put, ageing is the process of getting older.

It is easy enough for us to identify someone who is 'aged' and someone who is not. Visually speaking, an elderly person may have more wrinkles, or move more slowly, or their hearing may not be as good as it once was.

Ageing is a natural, physical process. Over time, our bodies accumulate damage and our organs suffer from wear and tear. This gradually results in a decrease in physical functioning, an increased risk of disease, and ultimately, death.[1]

It should not come as a surprise that the social changes which occur as a result of transition can bring about psychological changes as well. Getting older is associated with a myriad of life changes, all of which are accompanied by differing emotional processes. Some of these transitions might be positive, such as a well-earned retirement or the arrival of long-awaited grandchildren. Others, less so, such as the onset of illness or the death of loved ones.

What is harder to define is *when* ageing occurs. A traditional cut-off that many organisations and institutions use is the age of 65. But this number can be arbitrary, because ageing proceeds differently in individuals due to our genetic makeup, environment and lifestyles. Some individuals at the age of 65 are healthy and independent; others may already be affected by serious illnesses. Nonetheless, what is widely agreed upon is that, in the human species, ageing is inevitable, and so is its end result, death. Therefore, the journey of ageing is something every one of us has to take, whether we like it or not.

Ageing's Physical Effects and the Impact on Our Well-Being and Daily Functioning

Grace (not her real name) is a 73-year-old lady being treated for anxiety and depression. Premorbidly, she drove herself around and helped to ferry her grandchildren to school or classes. She cooked for her family on a regular basis and enjoyed exercising with her friends. Two years before we met, she developed worsening vision due to cataracts and had a near-accident while driving. She also fell twice at home. While she did not need to be hospitalized for her falls, she was observed in the A&E each time, and sustained bruises to her arms and legs. Her family hired a helper to assist her with chores, which meant that she cooked less while she recovered from her falls. She was also advised to stop driving until she could undergo an operation for her cataracts. As a result, she could no longer drive her grandchildren around.

As we get older, systemic changes occur in various parts of our bodies. The process starts out in a subtle and gradual manner from our thirties and forties, then speeds up as we approach our sixties and seventies. We lose muscle mass and skin tone. Our joints may weaken, and we develop aches and pains. We might lose some of our hearing or eyesight, and even our senses of smell and taste. Common health issues start to occur, such as hypertension, constipation, incontinence, and falls. This is excluding any other illnesses, stressors, or life transitions that might be ongoing simultaneously.

Another important physical change that occurs is in our brains. As we age, our brains shrink in volume. At the same time, changes to our blood circulatory system causes reduced blood flow to our brains. Both of these has a direct impact on our memory and ability to perform tasks, and this puts many of us at an increased risk of stroke and its complications.

Once we understand the physical effects of ageing, we can understand how this has an impact on our confidence and self-esteem, which in turns affects our lifestyle and level of independence. As in the illustration above, an older person may start to have difficulties with complex tasks that require sufficient cognition and input from sensory systems, such as driving, cooking, adapting to new technology, or exploring a new and unfamiliar place on their own. Being unable to perform such tasks as well as before can have an impact on an individual's level of confidence. To adapt to these difficulties, the older person may start to avoid them or increasingly rely on others for help. This then results in changes to their level of functioning and their independence.

Our Apprehension Toward Ageing

Grace grew more anxious about doing things on her own, fearing she would fall again or have another near-accident. She also became withdrawn and did not feel like cooking, even though there were opportunities to do so. She grew more reliant on the helper who had been hired to help her. She even stopped interacting with her regular group of friends. She described feeling unhappy with her current way of living. On the one hand, she understood why she had to make certain changes in her life. Some of these changes were only temporary, such as not driving until she had her cataract operation. Yet, she constantly compared herself to when she was younger, feeling that she was more capable and independent then. She lamented taking her health for granted in the past, and asked, "Why am I like this, doctor? Why can't I go back to the way I was?"

Ancient world mythologies are rife with references to immortality and the afterlife, and history records multiple accounts of individuals or groups of individuals striving for what seems to be unattainable — the search for eternal life. The ancient Greeks believed that consuming the mythical 'food of the gods' — nectar and ambrosia — could cure diseases, reverse ageing and make one immortal. The Bible's book of Genesis makes reference to the Tree of Life in the Garden of Eden, which grew fruit that could make one live forever. China's first emperor, Qin Shi Huangdi, was famously obsessed with immortality, though ultimately unsuccessful in his quest.

It is also inherently understood that such questors seek the secret to eternal life *with* eternal youth, unlike the Cumaean Sibyl of Greek mythology, who was granted a year of life for every grain of sand held in her hand, but ended up cursed by the god Apollo to live all those years without eternal youth. She ended up growing so old and shrinking to such a small size, that she could fit into a bottle, or so the legends said.

Even in our modern day and age, despite an implicit acceptance that an 'elixir of life' is unlikely to be found, scientists continue to conduct research to improve our understanding of why our cells and bodies age, and whether the process can be arrested, or even reversed. One area of particular interest is in telomeres (the end segments of chromosomes) and their role in ageing.

Outside of science and research, society as a whole continues to be fascinated by beings and creatures that are supposedly immortal because they capture our deepest desires to remain youthful, conquer ageing, and outwit death. Tolkien's elves, while not impervious to fatal injuries, did not age and could live for thousands of years. Vampires are equally fascinating (as the popularity of films and television series about them illustrates) because of their ability to stave off death and disease, have supernatural powers, and not age or die.

All of this means that for thousands of years, humans have raged against ageing and its inevitable end result, death. And we continue to do so, though perhaps in different ways than our ancestors. Some of us might seek treatments that purportedly reverse the effects of ageing (such as beauty treatments and Botox), others might become obsessed with being health-conscious and the latest diet or exercise trends. The fact that our society continues to rage against ageing means that certain labels also continue to be associated with becoming older. While some are positive, ('experienced', 'wise', 'golden years'), many are not ('useless', 'out of touch', 'dependent' and 'senile').

As a side note, there are differences in the way various cultures perceive ageing. Western cultures, which have a great global influence, lean toward a more negative perception of ageing and the elderly. Eastern cultures tend to view the elderly with great respect, such as including them in major family decisions, and enlisting grandparents to raise grandchildren. Singapore lies at a juxtaposition of these two differing worldviews, and it is not uncommon to see or hear examples of both.

When it comes to understanding why people have such an apprehension of ageing, it is important to understand that the process of ageing involves changes to our bodies, minds, and lifestyles, that are easily perceived as 'losses'. We may experience changes in our appearance, a reduction in our stamina and physical fitness, as well as our sexual health. We may find ourselves having to take multiple medications for health concerns, and losing our independence due to illness or hospitalisations. We might become replaced at work, or asked to retire. Our circle of support may grow smaller as our children embark on their own lives and raise their own families ('empty nest syndrome'), and our friends begin to pass on. Multiple 'losses' leads to a feeling of increased uncertainty about the future.

Loss is accompanied by grief. Grief itself is characterised by five stages: Denial, Anger, Bargaining, Depression and Acceptance. While not everyone will go through grief as they grapple with the process of ageing, some will. Those that do may go through all five stages, experience overlaps in stages, or even repeat stages as further changes occur.

As illustrated by Grace, some individuals will go through periods of grief as they come to a realization that their bodies and minds are not what they used to be in their younger days, or even prior to the crisis or turning point that for them, defines, ageing. Grace struggled and raged with this in her own way as she navigated the changes made to her lifestyle. She sought to find a balance between the changes in her body and her need for continued autonomy and self-reliance.

Another important psychological process to understand is what's known as Stage 8 of Erikson's stages of psychosocial development. Erik Erikson was a German-American psychologist and psychoanalyst who famously coined the term "identity crisis".[2] Erikson and his wife, Joan, developed a concept of healthy psychosocial development through an individual's life, starting from infancy. This theory is still used today to help patients and clients who experience mental health issues.

Stage 8 is theorised to be the final stage of psychosocial development, and it is experienced by individuals after the age of 60. In this stage, the basic virtue being developed is that of Wisdom. The psychosocial conflict at play is between Ego Integrity versus Despair. During this stage, individuals begin to reflect on their lives and begin to ask themself this fundamental question, 'Have I lived a meaningful life?'

Such existential thought occurs because as we age, our productivity declines and life gradually revolves around activities associated with retirement. We then start to contemplate our achievements. If we have perceived ourselves to have led a successful life, we develop Integrity. If we view our lives as unproductive or that we have not accomplished our life goals, Dissatisfaction and Despair set in. This would often then lead to feelings of depression and hopelessness.[2]

Ultimately, the apprehension each of us has toward ageing, and while we age, is normal. It is important to thus navigate the emotions associated with the process, in order to achieve peace of mind, even as the inevitable effects of ageing come upon us.

Ageing's Psychological Impact

Grace began to worry about her health excessively. She became extremely sensitive to every sensation in her body, and grew anxious that her health was deteriorating further (though there was no evidence that this was the case). She experienced palpitations and shortness of breath, which she interpreted to be signs of a heart attack, though her doctors told her that her heart was fine on several occasions. She began to sleep poorly because she was so worried about her health. Her family finally brought her to see a psychiatrist because she was tearful, and began to express thoughts that death was better than living.

Grace's example highlights a possible psychological impact that ageing can have on our mental well-being. The impact can also occur whether the changes of ageing are sudden (as in the case of a stroke) or gradual (as in Grace's case). What matters is that the events are *life-changing*.

And as part of having to deal with these life changes, individuals can develop increased levels of stress and frustration, and experience sadness and anxiety. Thus, it is not uncommon for the elderly to experience some level of anxiety or depression as they grapple with the different lifestyle that ageing brings upon them. Chief among these concerns is usually the fears of hospitalisation, disability and pain, taking multiple medications (which are often necessary), managing chronic illnesses, and increasing isolation as their circle of support diminishes.

Another aspect of ageing are the inappropriate strategies that people may turn to, to cope with their distress. Grace became overly preoccupied by health concerns, thinking that there were problems when there were none, and this resulted in excessive worries for her. On the flip side, other behaviours may involve denial and avoidance, where an individual might not acknowledge that there are any issues and not adjust their lifestyle accordingly to better manage their chronic conditions. They might even avoid seeing doctors or healthcare professionals completely.

Other maladaptive ways of coping could include turning to alcohol or substances (such as sleeping pills). In extreme cases, an individual can become suicidal, or they can begin to express thoughts that life is hopeless or has no purpose. Being in the elderly age group increases one's risk of suicide, and this is something that we should all be mindful of.

Related to the psychological impact of ageing is the physical change in our brains as we age. The normal and cumulative effects of brain shrinkage and reduced blood flow is a physical effect that has psychological consequents, namely, in the form of memory problems. We begin to forget minor things like where we placed our things, or taking our medications, or we may have difficulty recalling someone's name. When these cognitive impairments begin to affect our day-to-day functioning, professional advice and perhaps medication may be needed. As we become more absentminded and forgetful, we may also experience changes in our mood and a reduced tolerance for frustration. Further details on how to recognise the signs and symptoms of memory problems, and when to seek help, are available in the chapter on Dementia.

Getting Help

Grace received a short course of medication for her anxiety. She also saw a counsellor, who guided her through the psychological issues she was dealing with. With time, she grew to accept her "new normal", and could look back on her life with satisfaction. She eventually underwent a cataract operation, which allowed her to resume driving, albeit for shorter distances and only in the day time. She resumed cooking, and began to socialize as she did in the past. Life was beginning to take on new meaning once more.

One significant hurdle in helping an elderly person who is struggling with mental health issues is their own reluctance to seek help. There are several reasons why this could happen — the individual may have difficulty accepting that there is a problem, or have a stigma against being labelled, or there might be a complete lack of awareness that there are problems at all. In such instances, it is usually the family or significant other of the elderly person who first recognises these issues.

In order to overcome this hurdle, it is imperative for the elderly person's loved ones to engage with the individual in a sensitive manner, to gain trust and show support, before starting a conversation about mental health and seeking help. How each person achieves this varies depending on the dynamics of the relationship, but also involves awareness and openness on the part of the loved one approaching the elderly person in need. Sometimes, family members may turn to close friends of the elderly individual as a means of reaching to the person who needs help.

In Grace's case, she recognised that her anxiety was preventing her from having a normal daily life, aside from the limitations that ageing had brought upon her. It was this recognition that enabled her to be willing to seek help once her children also realised that she was suffering. Her self-awareness meant that she would engage better with her healthcare professionals, as well as make the necessary psychological adjustments in order to achieve her 'new normal'.

Another potential hurdle to an elderly person getting the help they need is navigating Singapore's rather complex healthcare system. It is important to identify what the healthcare needs of the elderly person are — do they need a psychiatrist? Or a geriatrician? Or a physiotherapist? Where mental health issues are obvious, as in Grace's case, psychiatric help would be warranted and sufficient. However, some individuals would have more complex needs, requiring a multidisciplinary approach with more than one specialist involved, and more than one allied health professional working with the elderly person.

Besides these, there are also multiple other avenues of support available in Singapore, including counsellors, psychologists and family therapists, who are accessible in the community through the government's Family Service Centres, through the restructured hospital system, and in private clinics.

One warning sign that makes seeking help of utmost importance and urgency is if the elderly person begins to experience thoughts of suicide, as in Grace's case, just before she sought help. As briefly mentioned in the previous section, the risk of suicide is increased in someone who is older. Other risk factors include physical illness, recent life crises, and social isolation.[3]

Hence, for the elderly individual struggling with the psychological impact of ageing, getting the help they need will benefit them in multiple ways — including helping them to regain some level of their former function, treat any mental health issues, as well as providing the awareness and insight to help them adapt to a new way of living.

Having realised that ageing was a reality, Grace decided that it was time to talk to someone about practical matters, like making a will and arranging for her end-of-life plans. She became rather lost with the vast amount of information available, finally she decided to get help from a lawyer.

End-of-life (EOL) planning is an important aspect of growing old, and it is a process best started by the elderly individual. To kickstart this process, one can do an Internet search, or talk to friends, or read information that is regularly available in our local newspapers. Sometimes though, as Grace found, the amount of information can be overwhelming and not specific to an individual's needs. This is where a lawyer, well-versed in such matters, and who knows the person well, can step in to tailor the process to the elderly person's needs, wishes, and based on their personal assets. Doctors enter the picture where there is a need for a medical certification or a medical assessment.

Details of EOL planning can be found in the next chapter by Dr Rachel Ng. Suffice to say, there are several aspects of end-of-life planning and care that should be addressed, preferably before the elderly person is too ill or incapacitated to do so.

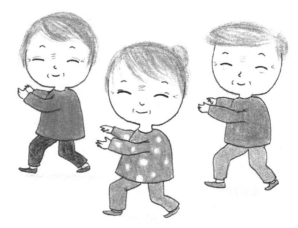

How Do I Safeguard My Mental Well-Being During the Process of Ageing?

After a year of treatment and counselling, Grace began to feel much better. Though she wasn't as involved in ferrying her grandchildren as before, she found other ways to spend time with them, such as having meals and taking them for outings (by taxi). Once her cataract operation was done, she started to volunteer at a nearby community centre, cooking meals for more needy elderly folks. In her spare time, she would meet up for lunch or tea with her close group of friends. She continued to exercise regularly — taking frequent morning walks, and doing stretches that her physiotherapist had taught her, so that she would remain limber and agile, and minimise her risk of falls. With help from her counsellor, Grace found ways of dealing with the changes in her life that she knew were associated with ageing. Even though more changes are likely to come as she grows older, Grace's perspective of the process and her response would probably be more positive than before.

The earlier sections of this chapter have described the potential psychological effects ageing can have on us. Some of these effects are unavoidable, such as the physical process of ageing itself. But some can be mitigated, which can help strengthen an individual's resilience through the process of ageing.

Being aware of the psychological impact of ageing is the first step to making the necessary adjustments in one's life and outlook on life. Self-awareness increases insight, which means difficult conversations (such as having to stop driving or make a decision about an operation) can be conducted with a clearer mind, and decisions can be made with more confidence. One other effect of awareness is that it enhances an individual's ability to express themselves, which is important for an older person, who may not be used to asking for help, or know how to voice their emotions and feelings.

Maintaining a robust social network is vital to building resilience as well. As we age, the natural tendency is for our network of support to become smaller and more limited, usually to our children or significant other. Our friends start to struggle with their own health problems, or even pass away. Our siblings face the same limitations. Nonetheless, keeping active in the community remains a crucial way for an elderly individual to remain connected, and feel relevant. This is where our local Senior Activity Centres, community centres and befrienders play a role in ensuring our elderly folks continue to get the support they need. Beyond that though, the individual needs to be motivated to maintain this social network for the benefit of their well-being. It is not uncommon for older individual to even serve in such settings, volunteering to cook for their peers or befriend folks who are even older than them.

An extension to remaining connected is the engagement that an older person needs to have in activities. Retirement is associated with aging. But retirement does not mean that the older person has to be idle. It is an opportunity to take up new hobbies, revisit old ones, and stimulate the mind in ways that it has not experienced before in the past. Local research has shown that certain activities promote mental well-being in the elderly and has positive effects on cognition; these include mahjong, gardening and listening to music.[4]

Other physical activities are equally important. Regular physical exercise, a healthy diet, cutting down on smoking and alcohol, and a proper night's sleep all contribute to promoting resilience, and help an older person to safeguard their mental well-being during the process of ageing.

Conclusion

Unlike the famous catchphrase of the Marvel Cinematic Universe's villain, Thanos, ageing *really* is inevitable. Naturally, so are the psychological adjustments necessary to cope with ageing and its physical effects. So rather than 'raging' against ageing, what matters is that each of us builds up our awareness, resilience, and psychological reserves. This will enable us to adapt and continue to maintain a positive outlook on our lives even in the midst of the uncertainties that ageing can bring about.

References

1.   Ageing and Health. World Health Organisation; 2021 Oct 4. Available at: https://www.who.int/news-room/fact-sheets/detail/ageing-and-health
2.   Erikson's Stages of Psychosocial Development. Wikipedia; 2022, Jan 14. Available at: https://en.wikipedia.org/wiki/Erikson's_stages_of_psychosocial_development
3.   Older Adults. Suicide Prevention Resource Center. Available at: https://www.sprc.org/populations/older-adults
4.   Kua EH. Colours of Ageing: 30 Years of Research on the Mental Health of the Singapore Elderly. Singapore: Write Editions (2018).

END-OF-LIFE PLANNING

Take Home Points

1. Although deliberate planning for our final days may not be a priority in our culture, it is necessary today more than ever, and better done earlier than later, as life is uncertain.
2. Planning ahead and sharing your preferences will enable your loved ones to carry out your wishes accordingly and with great clarity.
3. Organize your financial and legal documents and keep them in a safe place where a trusted family member or friend is aware of.
4. Consider your healthcare preferences and document an advance care plan.
5. Lastly, remember to write a will, make a CPF nomination and consider making a lasting power of attorney.

Mdm Yeo's younger sister, Dolly, was a 67-year-old single lady. Since their father's passing a decade earlier, Dolly had taken on the role as the main caregiver for their 90-year-old mother living with Alzheimer's disease dementia. Every sunday, it was usual for Dolly and her mother to take two buses to get to church where they would meet Mdm Yeo and attend morning worship service together.

Dr Rachel Ng Qiao Ming is an Associate Consultant in the department of Geriatric Medicine, and is currently practising at the Singapore General Hospital.

One Sunday morning, they were two hours late. Upon their arrival at church, Mdm Yeo noted that Dolly had significant pain over her right leg which made it difficult for her to walk. Dolly was taken to the Emergency Department where she was immediately admitted with severe pain from what was subsequently diagnosed as a right hip fracture.

During her first week of hospitalisation, Dolly developed fever with visual hallucinations. Subsequently, she was observed to have dangerously low oxygen levels with high carbon dioxide levels in her blood - despite a good course of intravenous antibiotics - requiring the extraordinary life sustaining measure of mechanical ventilatory support in the ICU. She was later diagnosed to have acute interstitial pneumonia - a rare condition that frequently leads to respiratory failure within weeks. Notwithstanding a total of 55 days of extraordinary life sustaining measures in the ICU, she did not recover and eventually passed on.

The family was at a loss. Neither of her older sisters expected their younger sister to be stricken so suddenly with an illness that took her life away. Throughout Dolly's hospitalization they were unsure as to what her wishes would be. She has not had any previous end-of-life conversations with them, and she could not communicate with them after becoming acutely ill, as she was kept intubated on mechanical ventilation. Thus, they had no choice but to make difficult decisions on her behalf and what they considered to be in her best interest based on what they knew about her.

Why is it important for me to start planning ahead for end of life?

Life is uncertain and death is inevitable. Dying well is rarely a coincidence, rather it results from choices made throughout life, and it is simply living well right up until the end. Although no one really wants to think about end of life, it is important to plan for the future so as to provide peace of mind for your loved ones, and help them to carry out your wishes when you are nearing end of life. There is no right or wrong time to have a conversation about your preferences for medical care, funeral arrangements or inheritance. It is just important to let your loved ones know your wishes, and you can save them from making difficult decisions-or worse still, wrong decisions on your behalf, without knowing what you would have wanted. By planning ahead and sharing your preferences, you can help your loved ones to carry out your wishes calmly, prepared with information, options and costs.

What does end-of-life planning entail?

End-of-life planning involves reflecting on and talking about:

- How you would want to be cared for at end of life
- Who you would want to make decisions for you if you lost your mental capacity
- How and where you would want your funeral to be conducted
- How you would want your assets to be managed after your death (i.e. life insurance/CPF nomination or will).

How should I get started?

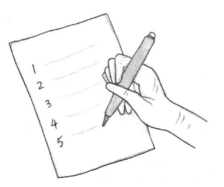

To get started, you can:

- Write a will
- Make a CPF nomination
- Make an advance care plan
- Make a lasting power of attorney
- Share your funeral wishes
- Organise, store and share important documents.

Who can make a will?

To write a will, you must:

- Be 21 years old and above
- Be of sound mind
- Make your will voluntarily without being forced or taken advantage of by someone else.

A will can be written by yourself. You may consult a lawyer if you want to make sure that your will is legally valid, or if your will is likely to be complicated. Muslims can make a will that is compliant with Muslim inheritance laws.

Why do I need to make a CPF nomination?

CPF savings do not form your estate and will not be covered under the will.

What's the purpose of making an advance care plan?

With aging, there is increased risk of developing strokes and dementia. Persons with these conditions find it increasingly difficult to exercise good judgement, solve problems and verbalize their preferences. Hence, they become less able to make sound financial and healthcare decisions.

When Mdm Mok's grandmother suffered a serious stroke, she realized how difficult it would be for her children to decide on treatment for her. She resolved that she would not want to put her own children through such an ordeal. She decided to have her medical preferences documented in an advance care plan.

If you cannot speak for yourself one day, who would you want to speak on your behalf? Would that person know what decisions to make? Would you know what your loved ones are thinking?

ACP seeks to address patient autonomy and promotes care that is consistent with the values of patients when they can no longer speak for themselves.

What are the 4 simple steps in advance care planning?

1. Think about it:
   — Consider what you would need to live meaningfully and comfortably and what would be important to you at end of life
   — In the event of extended illness, understand your prognosis, and consider your treatment options
2. Talk with loved ones and caregivers:
   — Discuss wishes and goals of care with close family and friends so they can understand
   — Consider having one or two trusted loved ones who can be your voice.
3. Put wishes into a plan:
   — Record and share decisions and wishes with appropriate individuals
   — Share and discuss these future healthcare choices with the attending doctor.
4. Review your preferences:
   — You can always change your mind after the plans are made.
   — If you change your mind, be sure to update the ACP documents and make new copies for the trusted parties involved.

How can I protect my interests with a lasting power of attorney in the event I lose mental capacity to make decisions for myself?

The Lasting Power of Attorney (LPA) is a legal document that confers upon one or more persons the authority to make decisions and act on the signee's behalf. The signee must be at least 21years of age to voluntarily make this appointment, should he/she lose the capacity to make his/her own decisions. A certified issuer must sign the LPA as a witness and certify that your loved one is aware of the implications of making an LPA. A certificate issuer can be a psychiatrist, a practicing lawyer or an accredited medical practitioner.

There are 2 types of LPA forms:

Form 1: A standard version that individuals use to grant general powers with basic restrictions to their donee(s).

Form 2: A version for those who have non-standard requirements and wish to grant customized powers to their donee(s). It is typically chosen by those who have larger and more complicated estates.

What are some considerations regarding funeral wishes that should be shared?

Share your funeral wishes according to this checklist:

Select a funeral service provider	Select someone to handle your funeral affairs	How the remains will be handled	Type of funeral service	Location of the funeral wake	Other preferences
▪ Inform family of a preferred funeral service provider so that they know who to contact for help when death occurs ▪ Consider buying a prepaid funeral plan from a funeral service, to reduce financial burden or stress when the time comes	Prior to your selection, consider: ▪ how well they can handle your funeral affairs ▪ whether they will make decisions that represents your wishes	▪ Burial ▪ Cremation ▪ Store ashes in a crematorium ▪ Store ashes at home ▪ Sea burial (ash scattering at sea)	▪ Christian ▪ Buddhist ▪ Muslim ▪ Hindu ▪ Non-religious	▪ Funeral parlour ▪ Church ▪ HDB void deck or multipurpose hall ▪ Pusara Aman Mosque (for Muslims only) ▪ Other facilities (please specify)	▪ Songs, hymns or music ▪ Prayer, poem or other readings ▪ Type of flowers ▪ Donation in your name to an organisation

How should I organise, store and share important documents?

Organise important legal documents according to these 7 categories:

Planning documents	Personal information	Financial accounts	Property & vehicles	Bills & payments	Digital assets	Others
1. Write a will 2. Make a CPF nomination 3. Make an advance care plan (ACP) 4. Make a lasting power of attorney (LPA) 5. Make an advance medical directive (AMD) 6. Share your funeral wishes	1. Your identification documents (NRIC and passport) 2. Birth certificate(s) 3. Marriage certificate(s) 4. Divorce certificate(s)	1. Bank accounts 2. Credit cards 3. Insurance 4. Loans 5. Investments 6. Safe deposit boxes	1. Residential property 2. Commercial property 3. Vehicles	1. Utilities (e.g. electricity, gas, water etc.) 2. Recurring payments (e.g. paid subscriptions for mobile, internet etc.)	1. Email accounts 2. Social media accounts 3. Online business accounts 4. Devices (e.g. laptop, phone, tablets etc.)	1. Pets 2. Other instructions

Put your important papers and copies of legal documents in one place and let a trusted family member, friend or lawyer know this location. These documents should be reviewed yearly as you may change your mind with time. It is fine to remove or add anything new and more importantly to ensure that your information is up-to-date. You could keep a file at home or consider storing important documents securely online with the My Legacy vault (https://www.mylegacy.gov.sg/) which allows you to add your loved ones as 'Trusted Persons' and grant them secure online access to your documents.

How My Legacy vault works

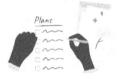

Simple guide to help you plan

Start with planning your will, lasting power of attorney, advance care plan, CPF nomination and funeral wishes.

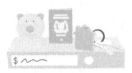

Keeping your information safe

Upload your documents to My Legacy vault for secure storage and share them with those you trust.

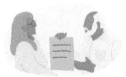

Make sure your family will be taken care of

Make it easy for your loved ones to access your plans and important information when they need to.

Figure 1.   What is My Legacy about? (Image courtesy of www.mylegacy.gov.sg)

Further Reading

End-of-life planning — My Legacy vault <https://www.mylegacy.gov.sg/vault/?redirect=/vault/>

John Dunlop, Finishing well to the Glory of God: Strategies from a Christian physician. (Illinois: Crossway, 2011), 12–13.

Advance Care Planning <www.aic.sg/care-services/advance-care-planning>

Office of the Public Guardian guide to LPA <https://www.msf.gov.sg/ opg/Pages/Home.aspx>

4

BARE ESSENTIALS FROM CRADLE TO GRAVE

Dr Lim Baoying

EXERCISE

Take Home Points

1. Exercise is not quite the same as physical activity; it is a subset of physical activity which tends to be of higher intensity and hence providing more health benefits.
2. Exercise provides multiple benefits such as the prevention of chronic medical conditions, healthier golden years and improving mental health.
3. Start low and go slow when starting an exercise regime, paying attention to the 'FITT' aspects of exercise.
4. To maximise the gains from exercise, do as much as possible, in terms of duration, frequency, intensity and variety.
5. Exercise is safe and confers benefits at all ages and physiological states in a woman's life.

What is exercise? Is it the same as physical activity?

Exercise is any planned, structured, repetitive bodily movements produced by your muscles that can increase your heart rate and burn calories. It is slightly different from physical activity which involves body movements at work (employed work or unpaid work, such as household

Dr Lim Baoying is a Registrar in Sport and Exercise Medicine, and is currently practising at the Changi General Hospital.

chores), travelling from one place to another, and/or during leisure, such as shopping. This definition was made by World Health Organisation (WHO)[1] in November 2020, in an attempt to provide clear guidelines for different populations and age groups to reap the overall, multiple benefits of exercise to one's body, mind and soul.

Do note that exercise tends to be of a higher intensity and will reap more health benefits, hence we encourage you to do exercise.

How are we doing in Singapore?

According to the last National Population Health Survey 2018/19,[2] 8 in 10 (80.1 percent) Singapore residents aged 18 to 74 years had sufficient (at least 30 minutes of at least moderate-intensity activities or equivalent for at least 5 days a week) total physical activity. However, only 1 in 3 (35.2 percent) exercises regularly (participates in any sports or exercise for at least 20 minutes per occasion, for at least 3 days a week).

Comparing the gender, a higher proportion of men exercise more regularly than women; and as we age, the prevalence of regular exercise also declines.

The hardest fact of all however, is that females constitute the largest population of obese individuals worldwide. Females with type 2 diabetes mellitus suffer more cardiovascular complications and mortality as compared to males.[3]

What are the benefits of exercise?

Exercise is truly the 'magic pill' that people have been seeking as a solution to longer lives in better health.[1,4] For the young, it serves as a gateway to a healthy adulthood, free from obesity and chronic medical conditions such as hypertension, diabetes mellitus and heart disease. For the adults, exercise is helpful in preventing the onset of those previously mentioned lifestyle-associated medical conditions, certain cancers such as breast and colon cancer, and can also help in the management of them. For the elderly, appropriate exercises can help improve their body composition, bone health, as well as prevent falls and fractures.

Exercise is also helpful in enhancing learning and thinking skills, reducing mental health symptoms of anxiety and depression, and slowing age-related decline in mental capacity.

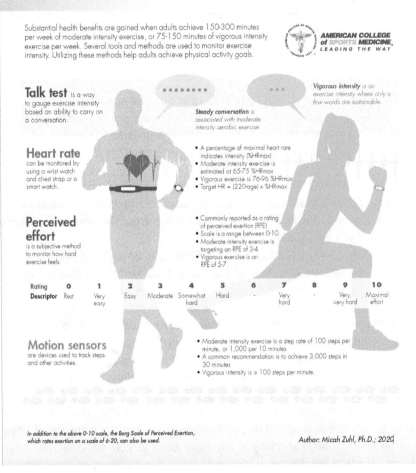

Figure 1. Tips for monitoring aerobic exercise intensity. (*Source*: American College of Sports Medicine.[5] Reprinted with permission.)

How should I get started?

At the start, your focus now should be on reducing sedentary behaviour. Moving more would confer more benefits. This first act can be easily taken by most people, for instance, by just reducing screen time and sitting down time.

As stated earlier, leisure time physical activity/exercise tends to be of a higher intensity and provides greater health benefits.

To begin, let's look at the different aspects of exercise, represented by the 'FITT' formula:

Frequency: how often do you engage in physical activity?
Intensity: how hard is your exertion level in the physical activity?
Time: how much time do you engage in the physical activity?
Type: what type of physical activity is performed?

The above-mentioned aspects of exercise are self-explanatory, except for *Intensity*. There are at least 3 commonly used methods of estimating your exercise intensity. Please refer to Figure 1 taken from the American College of Sports Medicine (ACSM).[5]

A widely used method is the ***Talk-Test***: light-intensity physical activity would allow one to sing/talk at the same time without difficulty; whilst moderate-intensity physical activity would cause the heart to beat faster than in light-intensity physical activity but still allow one to engage in a conversation. The latter is the recommended exertion level for most part of your physical activity. The other 2 methods are using a ***heart rate tracker*** during exercise and self-checking using a ***rating of perceived exertion (RPE)***.

A general rule of thumb is that 2 minutes of moderate-intensity activity is the equivalent of 1 minute of vigorous-intensity activity.

The FITT formula helps to provide a guide for the right dose of physical activity at different stages of one's life. Remember that the principle of 'start low, go slow' holds, especially if you have been largely sedentary, or have chronic medical conditions, which may cause you to question the safety of starting an exercise regime. There is largely no need for medical clearance if you are beginning with light-intensity or moderate-intensity physical activity, which do not exceed the demands of brisk walking or everyday living.

Have a look at the 2020 Physical Activity Readiness Questionnaire for Everyone (PAR-Q+)[6] to have a personalised guide as to how you should proceed onto taking the active first steps in your life.

Exercise is a beneficial habit to cultivate. To cultivate a habit, *frequency* is the most important aspect for you to start on. The more often you do an activity, the more likely it would become ingrained in you, and thus develop into a habit.

Duration (*Time*) and *Type* of exercise will be discussed with respect to age groups later.

What changes should I expect as I age?

Aging affects the body in multiple ways. Notably, those that would have a sizeable and noticeable effect on one's ability to exercise would be:[7,8]

- Reduction of lung capacity and chest wall flexibility such that it is harder to take in deeper and faster breaths.
- Lowered haemoglobin and haematocrit levels in red blood cells, such that the oxygen carrying capacity of the blood is reduced.
- Reduced heart pumping ability such that less blood volume is pumped out per cycle.
- Increase in blood pressure as a result of the reduction of arterial wall flexibility.
- Increased total blood cholesterol level with a reduction in the high-density lipoprotein (HDL), also known as the good cholesterol component.
- In the muscular system, there is a 40 percent reduction in the body muscle mass and 30 percent reduction of strength by the time a person hits the seventies. More notably, the lower body is affected to a greater extent than the upper body.
- 1 percent yearly decline in bone mass after the age of 35, and this rate increases to 2 to 3 percent decline with each passing year after menopause.

The flip-side is, once you start to exercise on a regular basis, some of these physiological declines can be reversed. You would be able to walk or run faster without feeling so breathless. You could possibly reduce or even stop your medication for diabetes mellitus, hypertension or high cholesterol because you don't need them anymore. Clinical studies have shown that older persons can become stronger and have reduced need for mobility aids as their bone and muscular strength improves.

What are the types of exercises I can do?

The main bulk of exercise for any person is aerobic activities.[1,4,5] We also refer to them as 'cardiovascular activities'. These are activities that engage the use of major large muscle groups in the body, and increase the breathing and heart rate. Activities include planned leisure-time exercise, transportation (such as walking or cycling), occupational work (especially if your job is not sedentary), household chores; basically the various physical movements that one usually performs daily. Some examples would include walking, jogging, cycling, swimming, games such as badminton, basketball, walking whilst playing golf, walking the dog, and household chores such as mopping the floor.

The simplest (leisure-time) exercise is brisk walking. The important point is that the walk should be done at a faster pace than a stroll in order for it to be considered as moderate-intensity. Do also take note that not all aerobic exercises are the same. Those that involve the lower half of the body, such as brisk walking and jogging would be considered as weight-bearing exercises. Weight-bearing aerobic exercises allow us to reap additional benefits such as increase in bone mineral density (BMD), and reduction of osteoporotic fractures.

However, for optimal health, we should add on other types of exercises as well. The requirements would vary according to individual needs.

Flexibility exercises are activities which help to maintain or improve the range of movements around a joint, and should be performed for all major muscle groups 2 to 3 days per week. Some examples would be static stretches and certain yoga poses. Each static stretch should be held for about 30 seconds, and repeated for 2 to 4 times per set. Such exercise is particularly useful for people with degenerative joint or back conditions such as osteoarthritis of the knees or lumbar spondylosis. A prominent symptom of degenerative joint condition is stiffness, which is brought on by period of inactivity. And yes, you guessed it right, being frequently active and stretching the soft tissues around the diseased joint is the counter movement for the symptoms.

Resistance exercise training or strength training are exercises that work our muscles to improve their strength and/or mass. They can be done against your own body weight (calisthenics e.g., burpees, push-ups, pull-ups, squats, lunges, planks), or by using equipment such as a resistance band, dumbbells, or even daily objects such as rice sacks or filled water bottles. Hence, even daily chores such as shovelling in the garden and carrying groceries can also count towards resistance exercise, but it would be hard to quantify the amount of exercise, compared to a session at the gym or one of calisthenics training. Ideally, everyone should perform resistance exercises, involving most major muscle groups, at least twice a week. The importance of strength training cannot be over-emphasised for the older individual in view of age-related muscle wasting. Being stronger will allow you to carry on with normal activities of daily living smoothly and also support your joints that are becoming worn out with age.

The last type of exercise is especially important for older individuals or anyone who is at risk of falls. We refer to them as balance activities, which serve to increase the strength of the legs, back and abdominal muscles and reduce the risk of falling, and the resultant risk of injury such as hip fractures. Some examples of these activities include Tai Ji, tandem walking (walking with your heel to toe) and practising standing from sitting on a chair, and they should ideally be performed at least thrice a week.

How much exercise is adequate?

It is important to keep active at any age, regardless of medical condition or physiological state. When there are limitations due to medical conditions (e.g., hypertension, heart disease, stroke) or physiological state (pregnancy, menstruation), and the recommended duration of physical activities cannot be met, just be as physically active as you can.

Prolonged inactivity is harmful to health. It could be simply working on the computer or laptop at home or at work; watching movies or Netflix; or video gaming. We put an arbitrary two hours per day of inactive screen time as physically harmful, especially to young children. Unhealthy weight gain, poor psychosocial skills and poor mental and physical development arise from such daily duration of inactive screen time. For every 30 to 60 minutes of being sedentary, try to schedule a break to walk around the office, climb stairs at home, or just do simple stretches, instead of remaining seated.

Table 1 provides actual leisure-time exercises recommendations for each age group. When these recommendations can be met, one can expect an improvement in cardiorespiratory and muscular fitness, bone and functional health, as well as reduction in the risks of non-communicable diseases, such as hypertension, diabetes mellitus, certain cancers, depression and cognitive decline.

Table 1.   Exercise recommendation for the various age groups.[1,3,4,10]

Age group (years)	Aerobic activities	Strengthening exercises	Others
5 to 17	F: daily	F: at least 3 days a week	Limit sedentary time, especially recreational screen time.
	I: moderate to vigorous	I: vigorous	
	T: ≥60min/ day	T: any duration (can be part of the 60min/day of physical activities recommended)	
	T: aerobic; e.g., running around in the playground, team ball games, badminton	T: bones and muscles strengthening; e.g., skipping rope, climbing, obstacle courses	
18 to 64 * includes patients who are suffering from cancer, hypertension, diabetes mellitus and HIV	F: almost daily	F: ≥2 days a week	Limit sedentary time
	I: moderate to vigorous	I: moderate to vigorous	Replace sedentary time with physical activity of any intensity for health benefits
	T: 150–300min / week (moderate intensity)/ 75–150min/ week (vigorous intensity)	T: any duration completing 2 to 4 sets of 8 to 15 repetitions of each exercise per session	Do more than recommended duration of moderate- and/or vigorous-intensity physical activities for additional health benefits
	T: aerobic; e.g., brisk walk, jog, cycle, swim, basketball or soccer games	T: muscle strengthening (all major muscle groups); e.g., lifting weights, body weight exercises, carrying groceries	

Table 1. *(Continued)*

Age group (years)	Aerobic activities	Strengthening exercises	Others
≥65 * includes patients who are suffering from cancer, hypertension, diabetes mellitus and HIV	F: almost daily	F: ≥2 days a week	Limit sedentary time
	I: moderate to vigorous	I: moderate to vigorous	Replace sedentary time with physical activity of any intensity for health benefits
	T: 150-300min/week (moderate intensity)/ 75–150 min/week (vigorous intensity)	T: any duration completing 2 to 4 sets of 8 to 15 repetitions of each exercise per session	Do more than recommended duration of moderate- and/or vigorous-intensity physical activities for additional health benefits.
	T: aerobic; e.g., brisk walk, jog, cycle, swim, walk during golf	T: muscle strengthening (all major muscle groups); e.g., lifting weights, body weight exercises, carrying groceries	Varied multi-component physical activities that emphasise functional balance and strength training at ≥ moderate intensity on ≥3 days a week to prevent falls and improve functional capacity

For children 5 to 17 years, it is crucial to cultivate the healthy habit of regular exercise. Active parents tend to encourage physical activity in their children as well. As the bodies of children and adolescents are still undergoing development, physical activities that aid in the development of mental resilience, social interactivity, musculoskeletal health and cardiovascular endurance are ideal. Unstructured play, team games, and outdoor activities such as hiking, kayaking, and obstacle course challenges are some examples of such activities.[10]

Once you hit your twenties, it is time for foundation building. Try out the different physical activities that suit your lifestyle. An enviable physique should not be the aim of your exercise, your overall health should be the priority. Defined muscles and killer abdominal walls are not the result of crunches alone, but the combination of a balanced diet and reduction of subcutaneous fats through physical activity. And if strength training has yet to be a part of your exercise regime, please start to incorporate one to two sessions of that per week to add to your peak bone mass and lean muscle bulk. Common pitfalls include unhealthy lifestyle habits like smoking, following fad workouts or diets, getting injured and having problems keeping up with and maintaining good nutrition and exercise.

In our forties we must work on preserving our strength and reducing the development of the middle-aged paunch. We will start to lose muscle mass more rapidly. Metabolic rate declines and hormonal changes from menopause can cause a build-up of visceral fats (also known as belly fats) as the decline in estrogen levels lays fat deep in our bodies after menopause. The scary fact is that visceral fats are not just unsightly, the amount of these fats also correlates with a woman's coronary health. Hence, exercise becomes even more important in combating these adverse changes to the body. A common pitfall faced by a woman at this stage is life's commitments. Smart time management and not overwhelming yourself are very important. Tell yourself that it is okay to ask for help.

As we progress into our sixties, we will need to be more careful— the risk of falls is higher after the age of 65. There is a five-time increase in the risk of death within a year of suffering a hip fracture. Strong muscles and bones, as well as good balance are needed to prevent falls and osteoporosis. Exercise will also help to reduce the risk of premature death from a chronic disease. There are multiple myths and misconceptions about physical activity in the elderly. It is never dangerous or too late to start exercising or continue being physically active. If you have chronic conditions such as heart disease, diabetes mellitus, hypertension, HIV infection or cancer, be as physically active as your condition allows for. You can check with your attending doctor on the type and level of physical activity appropriate for your condition and treatment plan. Of course, if you are unsure of anything when you are starting out in an exercise regime, you can ask for supervision from the sports trainers/health advisors in a nearby Active SG gym or Senior Activity Centre.

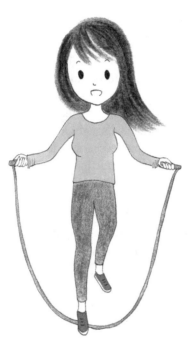

Is exercising during pregnancy safe? How often and what type of exercises should I perform?

A woman's body undergoes tremendous changes in pregnancy. Notably, the body fluid volume increases by 50 percent and that in turn, creates a 50 percent increase in the volume of blood pumped by the heart. Respiratory rate increases in view of the reduced lung capacity, just as body posture alters as a result of the foetus in the womb. These, and many more changes, are often too much for the pregnant woman to consider moving more than necessary, let alone pick up a new exercise regime.

Healthy pregnant women, with no medical or obstetric complications, should engage in at least 150 minutes of moderate intensity exercise per week, before, during and after pregnancy, as it is generally safe. Do not limit yourself to just aerobic exercises, but also include resistance and flexibility exercises for overall health benefits. This level of physical activity helps to prevent excessive weight gain, and onset of conditions such as gestational diabetes and pre-eclampsia.

There are certain conditions which would make exercise unsafe in a pregnant woman. Most are either pre-existing medical conditions, which are poorly controlled or severe disorders in the first place; or obstetric complications which would put maternal and/or foetal health at risk. Table 2[11] is not exhaustive and you should seek advice from your regular physician/ specialist in conjunction with your gynaecologist about physical activity. Further medical attention should be sought if there are warning signs such as chest discomfort, excessive breathlessness, giddiness, blood or amniotic fluid leak from the vagina, or painful contractions of the uterus.

Table 2.   Contraindications to exercise during pregnancy.

Absolute contraindications to exercise during pregnancy	Relative contraindications to exercise during pregnancy
Significant heart disease	Anaemia
Restrictive lung disease	Unevaluated cardiac arrhythmias
Severe anaemia	Mild to moderate cardiovascular disease
Uncontrolled systemic disorders including hypertension, thyroid disease and type 1 diabetes	Chronic bronchitis or other mild to moderate respiratory disease
	Malnutrition
Incompetent cervix including cerclage	Extreme underweight or eating disorders
	Morbid obesity
Intrauterine growth restriction	Heavy smoker
Multiple gestation at risk of preterm labour	History of extremely sedentary lifestyle
	Orthopaedic limitations
	Poorly controlled seizures
Unexplained vaginal bleeding or persistent second- or third-trimester bleeding	History of spontaneous preterm birth, premature labour, miscarriage or foetal growth restriction
	Recurrent pregnancy loss
Placenta previa after 26 weeks gestation	
Pre-eclampsia or pregnancy-induced hypertension	
Pre-term labour	
Pre-term pre-labour rupture of membranes (PPROM)	

If you have been regularly engaged in vigorous intensity exercise prior to pregnancy, you should continue with these activities during and after pregnancy. Women who are habitually engaged in vigorous intensity aerobic activity, or who are physically active before pregnancy, can continue these activities during pregnancy and the postpartum period. However, it is recommended that your heart rate should not be more than 90 percent of the maximal predicted for your age, in order to minimize the risk of low heart rate in the foetus.[3] Activities that involve physical contact, or carry risk of falls, injury to the abdomen, atmospheric pressure changes (for example, SCUBA diving or high altitude climbing) would not be advisable for the pregnant woman.

Avoid exercising while lying on your back (and especially on your right) after the first trimester due to the gravid uterus compressing the major vein returning blood to your heart. This could lead to dangerously low blood pressure, such that you could lose consciousness; the blood supply to the foetus could also be compromised.

How about exercising when having my menses?

Hormonal changes associated with the different phases of the menstrual cycle are generally considered the cause of a woman's fluctuating energy levels. We can attempt to divide the menstrual cycle into a typical 28-day cycle in order to explain things more simply.[12]

Days 1–7: the cycle starts when bleeding begins and oestrogen and progesterone levels are at their lowest. These levels start to rise during the period and the woman's energy level also goes up concurrently. Menstrual loss is messy, but with tampons, pads and menstrual cups, it is not difficult to continue exercising while having menstruation. The increase in blood circulation throughout the body during exercise helps to improve menstrual cramps and also reduces the abdominal bloating as a result of the increased motility of the intestines.

Days 8–14: Oestrogen levels peak for ovulation at mid-cycle and that rise in oestrogen level after the end of the bleeding is associated with an increase in energy level, this may lead to more physical activity. This is a good period of time to do strength training in view of the positive effect of oestrogen on muscular strength improvement.

Days 15–21: The fall in oestrogen level, concurrent with a rise in the progesterone level after ovulation causes a sluggish feeling that most women are familiar with. Getting physically active would help to counter this hormonal effect and allow you to feel more energetic.

Day 22–28: Both oestrogen and progesterone levels fall in the week before the next bleed, and your energy level would also decline further. Coupled with the onset of pre-menstrual symptoms (PMS) such as irritability, painful breasts and water retention, this can be a miserable week for many women. Exercise, at slightly lower intensity such as yoga or cycling, instead of running, would help to alleviate the symptoms while also keeping your body comfortable.

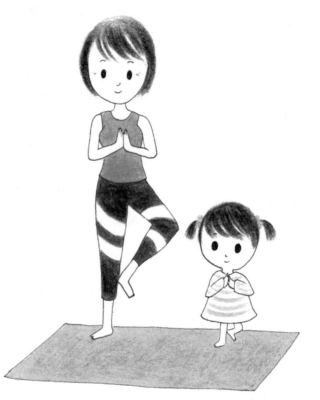

References

1. Physical Activity. World Health Organisation. Available at: https://www. who.int/health-topics/physical-activity#tab=tab_1
2. National Population Health Survey 2018/19. Ministry of Health, Singapore. Available at: https://www.moh.gov.sg/resources-statistics/reports/national-population-health-survey-2018-19

3. Pelliccia A, Sharma S *et al.* 2020 ESC Guidelines on sports cardiology and exercise in patients with cardiovascular disease. Taskforce on Sports Cardiology and Exercise in Patients with Cardiovascular Disease, European Society of Cardiology (ESC). *European Heart Journal* 2020; 1–80.

4. U.S. Department of Health and Human Services Physical Activity Guidelines for Americans, 2nd Edition. Available at: https://health.gov/our-work/physical-activity/current-guidelines.

5. Zuhl M. ACSM Tips for Monitoring Aerobic Exercise Intensity. American College of Sports Medicine; 2020. Available at: https://www.acsm.org/docs/default-source/files-for-resource-library/exercise-intensity-infographic.pdf?sfvrsn=f467c793_2.

6. 2020 Physical Activity Readiness Questionnaire for Everyone (PAR-Q+). Available at: http://eparmedx.com/wp-content/uploads/2013/03/January2020PARQPlus_Image.pdf

7. Rogers MA, Evans WJ. Changes in skeletal muscle with aging: Effects of exercise training. *Exercise and Sport Science Reviews* 1993; 21(1): 65–102.

8. Bemben MG, Massey BH, Bemben DA, Misner JE, and Boileau RA. Isometric muscle force production as a function of age in healthy 20- to 74-year-old men. *Medicine and Science in Sports and Exercise* 1991; 23: 1302–1310.

9. Garber CE *et al.* Quantity and quality of exercise for developing and maintaining cardiorespiratory, musculoskeletal, and neuromotor fitness in apparently healthy adults. *Medicine & Science in Sports & Exercise* 2011 July; 43(7): 1334–1359.

10. Singapore Integrated 24-Hour Activity Guidelines for Children and Adolescents 2020. Available at: https://www.ams.edu.sg/view-pdf.aspx?file=media%5c5924_fi_816.pdf&ofile=CPCHS+-+Singapore+Integrated+24+Hr+Activity+Guidelines+2020_Summary+(Final)+20200108.pdf

11. Lee R, Thain S *et al.* Perinatal Society of Singapore — Guidelines on Physical Activity and Exercise in Pregnancy; 2020 Jan 10. Available at: http://perinatal.sg/exercise.pdf.

12. Menstrual Cycle. Office on Women's Health. Available at: https://www.womenshealth.gov/menstrual-cycle.

DENTAL HEALTH

Take Home Points

1. Develop and maintain oral hygiene throughout life.
2. Learn the good brushing and flossing technique.
3. Identify a family dentist and make regular dental checkups before any dental problem arises.
4. Preserve the natural tooth structure for good aesthetics and function.
5. Seek early treatment for bleeding gums.

Women and Dental Health

Across all age groups, women are generally more concerned about oral health and are more likely to seek and receive professional dental care than men.

A woman's dental timeline begins in childhood and spans across young adulthood, motherhood, mid-life and finally the golden years. Each age group has particular characteristics. These are both physical, like hormone fluctuations during puberty, pregnancy and menopause, and lifestyle-related, such as eating habits and concerns about appearance.

Dr Loh Poey Ling is a Prosthodontist in private practice. She is also an Adjunct Associate Professor in the Faculty of Dentistry in the National University of Singapore.

Dr Lieu Yen Tung is a Dental Officer in the National Dental Centre.

The short discussions here highlight some common dental issues that are likely to be of interest and concern throughout a woman's lifetime. Certainly, some of these issues are not just specific to women.

Childhood to Young Adulthood

The cycle of milk and permanent teeth development can cause worries in parents and growing children.

My 3-year-old still drinks milk from the bottle and will suckle on milk to go to sleep. Is it ok?

A child should not go to bed with a filled milk bottle. This can cause decay in the child's teeth. Try swapping milk in the bottle to plain water if the child is unwilling to let go of the bottle. Honey water or any sweetened drink is not a good choice. You must ensure that the child's teeth have been brushed before sleep.

When should I bring my child for their first visit to the dentist?

It is recommended for a child to see a dentist when their first tooth erupts. It is important for the child to be comfortable in a dental setting. Even if the child is not receiving treatment at such a young age, having the child exposed to being in a dental clinic will familiarise the child with the sights and sounds in this foreign setting. Bring your toddler along to your next visit with the dentist, make it a pleasant outing!

Are there other important things I should note when taking care of my child's teeth?

Limit the frequency of snacking in children. It applies to adults like us too! It is not only sweet candies that can cause decay. Savoury crackers, bread or any food that remains on the surface of our teeth for a prolong period of time will cause decay.

We can help our children brush their teeth till they can brush their own teeth independently (around age 6 to 7). When the first tooth erupts, we can start using a clean, damp washcloth or a finger brush to gently wipe the tooth and the tongue after meals. When there are more teeth and the child can accept a toothbrush in the mouth, start brushing with a tiny smear of tooth paste. It is recommended that a rice-grain size amount of toothpaste be used in children under 2 years old. With older children, we can increase to a small pea-sized amount of toothpaste when brushing their teeth.

Make sure they do not swallow toothpaste when brushing their teeth. If the child tends to swallow the toothpaste, use a fluoride free toothpaste until s/he can follow instructions.

My child fell down and an entire tooth dropped out. What should I do?

It is important to establish if it is a baby tooth or a permanent tooth that has dropped out. A child below age 6 is not likely to have upper permanent teeth in the mouth yet.

If it is a baby tooth, DO NOT put the tooth back into the socket it dropped out from. If it is an adult tooth, it is strongly encouraged to put the tooth back into the socket as soon as possible.

Understandably, it might be hard to distinguish the correct direction to place the tooth back into the socket. If you are not confident of placing the tooth back into the socket it came out from, do the following:

1) Pick up the widest part of the tooth that is white in colour, try to avoid touching the yellow conical shape portion of the tooth.
2) Place the dislodged tooth in a cup of milk or into a cup that contains some of the child's saliva.
3) Immediately take the child to visit a dentist or an A&E department with the retrieved tooth.

If your child plays a contact sport, it is highly recommended that they wear a mouthguard while playing. This is to protect the teeth and reduce the risk of the trauma to the teeth.

My daughter's milk teeth are loosening already but she says none of the boys in her kindergarten class have shaky teeth.

All girls and boys have a similar set of baby and permanent teeth. Most of the 20 baby teeth (deciduous teeth) erupt by age 3, and at age 6, the first permanent molars start erupting behind the last deciduous molar. Each child has a different rate of growth and the same applies to the timing of tooth eruption and shedding (exfoliation).

Children go through the mixed dentition stage from ages 6 to 12 where both baby and permanent teeth are present in the mouth. Permanent teeth erupt simultaneously while the deciduous teeth exfoliate. The first milk teeth to exfoliate are the lower incisors followed by the upper incisors. Sometimes, permanent incisors take a while to show up and this worries parents. It's best to just let nature take its course and wait calmly.

There are times that the permanent tooth erupts through the gums behind the milk tooth. When this happens, the milk tooth will usually become shaky and exfoliate naturally. If the child has difficulty eating in this situation, a dentist can help to remove the milk tooth.

In rare situations, the permanent successor does not develop in the jaw. Please seek dental consultation if no successor erupts through the gums three to six months after the milk tooth has exfoliated. Radiographs (x-ray film) will be taken to check on the developing teeth in the jaw bone and if it is a condition of congenitally missing teeth, the dentist will monitor the child and choose the best timing of the treatment. This might involve braces (orthodontics) and prosthesis to replace the missing tooth/teeth if necessary.

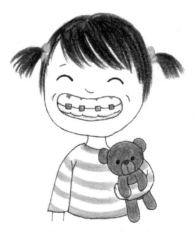

My 4-year-old child has crooked and overlapping teeth. Should he start braces treatment now?

When milk teeth overlap, permanent teeth have a high chance of misalignment when they erupt. Typically, braces (orthodontic treatment) will start only after all the milk teeth are replaced by permanent teeth, at around age 12 or even later.

In some situations, when moderate to severe growth discrepancies at an earlier age are diagnosed, interceptive treatments may be recommended earlier to modify the growth of the jaw in order to simplify future treatments.

Is it necessary to remove the wisdom teeth?

Our third molars are commonly called wisdom teeth. They normally erupt around 18 years of age. A teenager may experience some discomfort in the back of the lower jaw when the tooth is erupting. If the alignment of the wisdom tooth is upright and good, and the jaw bone has enough space to accommodate the tooth, it will erupt uneventfully and function well with the opposing wisdom tooth just like the first and second molars. Extraction is not required unless it is not properly cleaned and begins to decay later in life.

In the process of eruption, a soft tissue tag covering the tooth may become infected due to food debris accumulation or trauma from the opposing tooth. There could be pus formation causing swelling of the face and severe pain. Treatment usually involves removing the wisdom tooth, or simply removing the soft tissue tag and leaving the wisdom tooth to erupt — if it is not impacted.

A wisdom tooth that is tilted and stuck behind the second molar is called an impacted wisdom tooth. This commonly occurs in the lower wisdom teeth. In such instances, removal is recommended. This reduces the risk of decay in the second molar root surface, which the wisdom tooth is jammed against.

Some wisdom teeth are deeply embedded in the jaw bone and not exposed to the oral environment. These teeth may be left alone. It is recommended to have periodic x-ray checks for bone changes around the buried tooth.

I am 25 years old and my impacted wisdom tooth has not given me any problems. Why should I remove it? Will my cheek collapse and affect my appearance after the removal?

The impacted wisdom tooth usually traps food that cannot be properly cleansed on your own. This can cause a large decay in the root of the tooth in front of it, resulting in severe toothache. This situation often occurs later in life, after 40 years of age. Removal of an impacted wisdom tooth will eliminate the food trap and reduce the decay risk. Cleaning of the last tooth in the back of the mouth then becomes easier.

A study found that older individuals have a greater risk of postoperative complications from impacted wisdom tooth removal. The risk is also higher among women.[1] The author thus recommended surgical removal of impacted mandibular third molars before the age of 24 years, especially for female patients.

The removal of a wisdom tooth will not cause changes in facial appearance. However, there will be some swelling for a few days after the procedure.

Will removal of the wisdom tooth cause damage to the nerve?

The oral surgeon removing the wisdom tooth will have radiographic assessment of the relationship between the nerve and the tooth. The nerve will be protected during the surgery. Most cases of surgery to remove impacted wisdom teeth are uneventful, with very little or no numbness experienced after the anaesthesia for the surgery wears off.

In some unfortunate cases, if the nerve is very close to the wisdom tooth, it may get stretched, bruised or crushed during the surgery. If this is the case, prolonged numbness and altered sensation could be experienced after the surgery. The injured nerve usually repairs itself and recovers between 8 weeks to 6 months. However, as mentioned, the incidence of such injuries is low.

Cases of permanent nerve damage are extremely rare, but these will result in permanent numbness.

I don't like the look of my teeth. The colour is too dark and they are not straight. I'd like movie star teeth. In fact, I'm thinking of putting veneers on my teeth. Is it a good treatment?

There are two problems with the teeth in this question here. The colour and the alignment.

The discoloration of teeth may be extrinsic which is only on the surface. It could be caused by food stains, ineffective brushing or bacterial plaque accumulation on the tooth. All these can be easily cleaned up and polished to regain the nice sparkle of natural teeth. Teeth whitening, or bleaching can then be done non-invasively to further brighten the teeth.

However, intrinsic discoloration of the teeth might be caused by certain drugs or chemicals taken during the formation of the teeth. This cannot be polished away. Veneers are only indicated in such cases — when professional bleaching doesn't achieve the desired results.

Mis-alignment or crooked teeth will be best corrected by orthodontics. Veneers are not recommended as the first line of treatment in most cases.

Straightening misaligned teeth (orthodontic tooth movement) takes at least 18 months. In complex cases, this can extend to over 2 years. There are cases where misaligned teeth need to be corrected in a short time. Veneers or crowns may be considered. However it might compromise the desired aesthetic outcome. Long term implications such as gums disease and risk of tooth decay must also be taken into consideration.

Pregnancy and Motherhood

When women become pregnant and enter into motherhood, dental issues may arise due to hormonal changes.

Am I at an increased risk of gingivitis during pregnancy?

Yes, gingivitis may be exacerbated due to hormonal changes during pregnancy. However, gingivitis and periodontal disease do not simply occur overnight nor are they caused by pregnancy.

When there is an accumulation of dental plaque and calculus (tartar) which contains bacteria, the gums will become irritated and this gradually results in inflammation. Subsequently, the gums start to bleed. Treatment is in the form of professional cleaning of the teeth and maintaining good oral hygiene — habits like brushing and flossing daily. Of course, this has to be accompanied by regular dental visits for professional cleaning to maintain a healthy oral environment.

My grandmother says that I will lose a tooth with every child born. Is it true?

This is not true. Carrying a child to term and delivering it does not cause a woman to lose her teeth.

In a situation where a woman has untreated gum disease (periodontitis) before pregnancy, it is possible that some teeth will loosen and that the gums will swell during pregnancy. Eventually some teeth could even be lost during or after pregnancy. Pregnancy can amplify the effects of pre-existing periodontal disease.

There have been swellings appearing at the gums between my teeth during pregnancy. Should I be concerned? My dentist told me that I don't have gum disease.

These soft tissue swellings are known as pregnancy epulis. They are benign tissue swellings that often recur during pregnancy but resolve spontaneously after pregnancy. Some individuals choose to have them removed as the swellings affect their smile aesthetically.

TIP: It is essential to maintain good oral hygiene habits before, during and after pregnancy to prevent tooth loss and decay. Regular cleanings can be done by a dentist even when pregnant.

More information is available online from the European Federation of Periodontology sources listed in the References section.[2,3]

What should I do to make my baby's teeth strong during pregnancy?

Folic acid is a widely recommended supplement for all pregnant women. It helps prevent birth defects and ensures healthy development. It is found in green leafy vegetables such as spinach, kangkong, broccoli, cabbage and chickpeas.

Calcium and phosphorous are important for the development of strong teeth. Calcium is found in dairy products such as milk, yogurt and cheese. Phosphorous is generally found in foods which are high in protein, such as meats, nuts, beans and dairy products.

Vitamin D helps us retain calcium and phosphorous in our bodies. It is an essential vitamin to ensure healthy bone development and growth. Vitamin D can be obtained through food such as oily fish (salmon, tuna, fish oil etc.). In addition, exposure to sunlight helps our body produce Vitamin D naturally, although excessive exposure to sunlight is not recommended.

A well-balanced diet that includes nutritious foods will help strengthen not only the teeth, but also ensure the development of a healthy baby.

Middle Age

As women approach menopause, dental issues may arise due to hormonal changes.

I have bleeding gums. It was bad during pregnancy, so I thought it was due to hormonal changes. Now, even though I am no longer pregnant, my gums are still bleeding. Why?

Bleeding gums is a sign of gum disease. It is not a disease specific to women. The bacteria in the accumulation of plaque and calculus around your teeth can irritate the gums and cause inflammation of the gums. This results in the bleeding. When left untreated, it will progress to bone loss and eventually tooth loss.

Proper brushing and flossing daily are the best methods to prevent the accumulation of plaque around the teeth and below the gums. The plaque that is not removed will harden to become calculus. Unfortunately, it is not possible for you to remove it on your own at home using toothbrush and dental floss.

Routine, six-monthly scaling and polishing of teeth can reverse the bleeding gums condition in gingivitis, but left untreated, gingivitis can develop into advanced gum disease known as periodontitis. The treatment of periodontitis requires deep cleaning in close intervals at the beginning. Some cases may require more advanced treatment procedures to save the teeth.

My dentist told me that I am clenching and grinding my teeth and I have TMD. What is it exactly?

TMD is the abbreviation of Temporomandibular Disorder. There are different categories of this disorder. It most often presents as headache and pain affecting the muscles involved in chewing. The other categories involve the internal derangement or degeneration of the jaw joints.

The pain in TMD may be mild with some discomfort or severe pain that affects daily life. It appears that women are more affected by TMD than men.

Some self-help tips while you are seeking proper professional treatment are: avoid hard food, extreme jaw movements such as wide yawning, singing loudly and deliberate stretching of the lower jaw. Applying a heat or cold pack may also help relieve the discomfort.

I recently experienced pain in my molar whilst chewing on it. I was told I have a cracked tooth. What will the dentist do to help me?

The problem of pain in a tooth when biting might be the result of a crack in the tooth. There could also be other causes. The dentist might place a metal band around the tooth. If this is able to stop the pain immediately, it confirms the tooth has a crack.

The treatment for a cracked tooth depends on how deep the crack extends and the condition of the pulp of the tooth. If the crack is shallow, a crown for protection of the tooth will be used to slow or stop the crack from propagating.

In the case of a deep crack, the pulp may already be violated with bacterial infection. This can potentially cause severe spontaneous pain in the tooth. Root canal treatment will be required, followed by a crown to protect the tooth. In most cases a root canal specialist is needed to assess the depth of the crack to see if the tooth is worth saving.

A mouthguard will be recommended to protect your other teeth from cracking.

My cracked tooth could not be saved, now it has been extracted. What are the different ways to replace my missing tooth? Can I choose not to replace it?

Depending on which tooth is lost, there are various possible treatments, namely implant, denture or a bridge. If the missing tooth is not visible when smiling and you are able to eat comfortably with many remaining pairs of opposing teeth, not replacing the tooth is an option. For example, a wisdom tooth is not usually replaced if it is lost. Some missing second molars are not replaced also.

However, not replacing a missing tooth has a risk. The adjacent teeth might start to drift into the space of the missing tooth over time. If the arrangement of the teeth is favourable, the drifting may be minimal and not noticeable and chewing function not affected badly.

Of course, if the missing tooth is in the visible zone, the appearance of the smile will be affected.

It is prudent to discuss the need for replacement and the various options of replacement with your dentist.

The Golden Years

As women enter their golden years, loss of bone density could cause some dental issues.

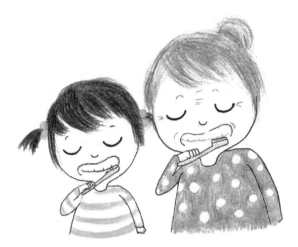

I was diagnosed with osteoporosis and I will be receiving injections for the treatment. I was told to see the dentist before the injection. Why?

It is for a thorough check-up of all teeth. Extracting teeth in individuals receiving osteoporosis treatment is best avoided. The drugs for osteoporosis treatment alter the way cells maintain healthy bone. The healing capacity of bone will be reduced. The dental check-up will hence identify potential dental problems and recommend treatment before starting the osteoporosis treatment e.g. teeth that require extraction.

It is important to maintain good oral health at all times and take care of any dental problems before they flare up.

My mouth is feeling very dry lately, food tastes different. What can I do?

Dry mouth or xerostomia occurs when the salivary glands are not producing enough saliva to keep the mouth wet. There are many possible causes for this condition.

It may be associated with medications for depression, high blood pressure, anxiety, muscle relaxants and many others. Diabetes, radiation treatment for head and neck cancer, and autoimmune disease like Sjogren's syndrome can also cause dry mouth. Ageing itself is also a possible cause as many older people experience dry mouth as they age.

An altered sense of taste is called Dysgeusia. It can be caused by dry mouth. There are many other associated contributing factors such as medications, chemotherapy, post nasal drip and smoking. Hormonal changes during pregnancy can also cause dryness in the mouth.

Inform the doctors about your dry mouth and altered taste problem. Sometimes change of medications can help improve the condition. Mouth rinses designed for dry mouth can also be effective.

Ensure that you are maintaining good oral hygiene habits such as proper brushing and flossing after every meal. Avoid snacking; keeping the mouth moist with mouth rinse or by sipping water frequently. The dry mouth condition predisposes the teeth to higher incidence of decay. Regular visits to the dentist for professional cleaning and application of topical fluoride is important.

Seek medical help to check and identify the underlying causes of an altered taste sensation and dry mouth.

I have had an ulcer in my mouth for many weeks. It does not hurt. I don't go for regular check-ups. Can I just leave the ulcer to heal by itself?

See a dentist as soon as possible. An ulcer that does not heal or hurt within the span of 2 weeks can be a sign of a malicious disease.

My mother has dementia and I am caring for her. What do I need to do for her oral health?

A person who has maintained good oral hygiene habits may be able to continue to clean their teeth in the early dementia stage. A caregiver will have to check for proper brushing. Ensure she goes for routine dental visits so that small problems can be resolved.

At home, remind her to brush her teeth in the morning and before bed. Flossing may be difficult if she is advanced in age, but it is encouraged if she can still manage. A caregiver will need to check that the cleaning is being carried out effectively. Very often, food particles may be left on the tooth surfaces, in between the teeth or under the denture even after brushing or rinsing.

Water irrigators and other small tools like interdental brushes can also be used to clean in between the teeth. Having a damp washcloth for wiping the gums and areas hard to reach by a toothbrush will be helpful. Please seek dental advice for the appropriate recommendations.

If she has a denture, remind her to remove it after every meal and clean it by brushing with a denture brush. Then soak it in water overnight. Denture cleanser solution is a good aid in keeping the dentures clean but brushing the denture properly with a denture brush is still important before and after soaking the denture.

It is important to be attentive with dementia patients who wear dentures. The elderly may misplace the denture after removing it for cleaning purposes. It may also be thrown away accidentally if the dentures are removed during meal.

Conclusion

As we journey through life, our dental needs and demands change. The one important thing to remember is to maintain our oral health. Keeping our teeth and gums healthy will help us move gracefully through life. A good set of natural teeth or functional dentition is a great asset to have, especially in one's golden years . Quality of life will be vastly better for those who have consistently maintained their oral health than for those who unfortunately have lost many teeth.

References

1. Blondeau J and Daniel NG. Extraction of impacted mandibular third molars: postoperative complications and their risk factors. *J Can Dent Assoc* 2007 May; 73(4): 325. Available at: https://pubmed.ncbi.nlm.nih.gov/17484797. PMID: 17484797.
2. Figuero E and Sans M. Women's oral health during pregnancy. European Federation of Periodontology. Available at: https://www.efp.org/fileadmin/uploads/efp/Documents/Campaigns/Oral_Health_and_Pregnancy/Reports/womens-oral-health.pdf.
3. Oral health and pregnancy FAQ. European Federation of Periodontology. Available at: https://www.bsperio.org.uk/assets/downloads/Oral_health_and_pregnancy_FAQ.pdf.

DEPRESSION AND SUICIDE IN WOMEN

Take Home Points

1. Depression is a real illness, it is not in your mind.
2. Depression is treatable.
3. You do not have to fight depression alone, help is available.
4. Medication is not the only treatment for depression, ask your care provider about options if you are not comfortable with medication.
5. Being depressed does not make you weak.

The gender gap is very real when it comes to depressive disorders. Women are nearly twice as likely as men to be diagnosed with depression. Suicide, however, is more common in men. According to statistics from the Samaritans of Singapore (SOS), 70 percent of completed suicide cases are male. Notably, this does not take into account the number of attempted suicide cases.

Rising mental health issues among women have been a trend in recent years, and part of this could be due to the increasing awareness around the

---

Dr Kamini Rajaratnam is a Consultant Psychiatrist, and is currently practising at the Better Life Clinic.

existence of mental disorders. It would be simplistic to assume that the differential sex ratio is merely due to increased help-seeking behaviour in women. A myriad of other reasons have been postulated for this; from the differential acknowledgement and high rates of completed suicide in men, to the biological mechanisms resulting from hormonal effects on the brain, to the epidemiological and social risk factors of motherhood, and increased risk of sexual and domestic violence and prejudicial treatment, both in the community and in the workplace, just to name a few.

The focus of this chapter is to define what depression is and outline what it can look like, as well as when and how to get help. Depression is a biological illness. Brain chemistry plays a significant role as depression is correlated with low levels of serotonin, norepinephrine and dopamine (neurotransmitters in the brain). Fortunately, this is also what makes it so treatable as well, as there is an arsenal of antidepressant medications that can help to correct this neurotransmitter imbalance. There is a very common misconception that depression can be fought or overcome using our minds. While mild forms of depression are very amenable to psychotherapeutic treatment methods, a trained mental health professional is still required to administer them. Unfortunately, the predominant narrative that is thrown at depressed women is to 'snap out of it' and 'be strong' through their ordeal. This causes a lot of guilt when they cannot feel better on their own, as well as reluctance to reach out to a mental health professional for treatment. This is commonly seen in the post- or prenatal population, as they are especially susceptible to mood and anxiety disorders. Newly minted mothers may receive conflicting messages that they should be grateful for their pregnancy/baby and that feeling otherwise shows one is a bad mother. This is simply not true. There are always help channels available to gather more positive thoughts for themselves and their baby.

What are some myths about depression?

Myth	Fact
Depression is all in your mind and you can get over it without help.	Depression is a biological illness. However, as its effects are felt on the way you think and feel, it is often not perceived as a medical illness.

(Continued)

Myth	Fact
Depression is incurable.	Depression is very treatable, with psychotherapy, medication or a combination of both.
Depression is a sign of weakness and a choice.	Being depressed is no more a choice than being diabetic or hypertensive. It is not a sign of weakness, and on the contrary the patients I have treated with depression, have displayed nothing short of superhuman strength throughout their fight with depression.
Depression is caused by circumstances. If nothing is going wrong in your life, you should not be depressed.	Depression is multifactorial. While external circumstances can cause depression, other factors such as genetics, an altered brain chemistry and the environment all play a role in the development of the illness.
If I am depressed and I seek help, I have to take an antidepressant medication.	Not everyone with depression needs antidepressant medication. In mild cases, psychotherapy alone and lifestyle changes help tremendously.
Depression will just go away.	Many people with depression do not reach out for help until many years after the onset of the illness. Depression requires treatment and the earlier you get it, the quicker you recover and the better your prognosis.
Depression is just feeling sad.	Depression is very different from normal feelings of sadness. Unlike the latter, depressed people have prolonged periods of fatigue, low motivation, loss of interest in usual

(Continued)

(Continued)

Myth	Fact
	activities, change in eating or sleeping patterns, physical aches and pains, feelings of loneliness, emptiness, worthlessness, anxiety, anger, and irritability. Individuals living with depression are more likely to experience suicidal thoughts. This is very different from normal feelings of sadness.
Talking about my feelings will make me feel worse.	Talking about your feelings allows you to have an outlet, receive validation and find solutions in a safe, non-judgemental space.

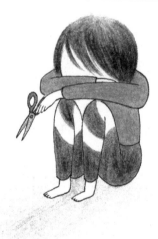

What are the signs and symptoms of depression?

1. Feeling sad and empty all the time.
2. Having difficulty falling asleep, staying asleep and early morning waking.
3. Having decreased or increased appetite/comfort eating.
4. Losing interest in activities you previously enjoyed.

5. Feeling easily irritated, frustrated and triggered by small things that did not previously bother you.
6. Having trouble concentrating at work or at home.
7. Feeling tired and lethargic constantly.
8. Having feelings of hopelessness, worthlessness and guilt.
9. Having thoughts of suicide.
10. Waking up in the morning and feeling very overwhelmed, unable to carry on with your day and wanting to stay in bed/sleep more.
11. These symptoms affect your functioning at work or at home.

Where can I get help if I am depressed?

If you are feeling suicidal, the Samaritans of Singapore (SOS) hotline at 1-767 is a good number to call immediately for assistance. It is a 24/7 hotline manned by trained counsellors.

Other avenues of help:

1. Polyclinics, General Practitioners: primary healthcare physicians are able to screen and treat simple cases of depression. They are also able to put out referrals to a psychiatrist or psychologist if necessary.
2. Psychologists, counsellors: provide supportive counselling and psychotherapy.
3. Psychiatrists: help to diagnose and formulate a treatment plan and assess if there is a need for medication.

What are the lifestyle changes that can help prevent depression and burnout?

An important part of the psychopathology of mental health disorders is an exaggerated stress response. A healthy stress response is protective and forms the basis of us being able to fight or flee from perceived threats. However, in chronic stress, the stress response becomes exaggerated and the long-term effects of this on our body are far ranging, from the gastrointestinal system, to the cardiovascular and immune system. It is therefore essential to keep our stress levels in check to prevent a chronically exaggerated stress response.

How do we do this?

1) Incorporate regular relaxation into your daily routine

- Yoga
- Mindfulness-based stress reduction
- Meditation
- Journaling: listing down what one can be thankful for, stream of consciousness free writing, writing down 'what went right', visualising scenarios, musical therapy and unsent letter-writing.

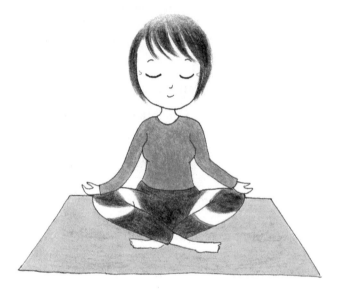

2) Optimise nutrition for mental health

- Gut health: regular intake of probiotics
- Omega 3
- Nutritional deficiencies: Zinc, Iron, Vitamin B12, Vitamin D, Magnesium
- Focus foods: Leafy greens, oily fish like salmon, eggs, dark chocolate, spices (turmeric, cinnamon), green tea, good fats, whole grains, legumes, nuts

What to avoid: Sugar, processed/refined food, alcohol, pesticide, hormones, antibiotics.

3) Sleep

- Regular sleep and wake times
- No electronics/screens 2 hours before bed
- No alcohol/large meals in the evening
- Cut off caffeine after mid-day

- No exercise 3 hours before bedtime
- Avoid long afternoon naps
- Wind down routine 1 hour before bedtime
- Use room only for sleeping/sex.

4) Exercise

- Relieves stress
- Improves memory
- Boosts mood
- Enhances sleep.

5) Connect with others

- Find your support network
- Connect with friends and family regularly
- Social connection: volunteering, organising virtual events
- Connect with your partner/children.

6) Take breaks from the news

- Stay informed but do not be overwhelmed
- Check on the news just once or twice a day
- Avoid too much exposure to the news cycle
- Take a break from social media.

7) Additional tips to help regulate your emotions

- Refocus attention onto what is positive in your life or day
- Reframe negative situations to see the positive in them
- Adjust your self-expectations. You do not need to function at 100 percent of your capacity all the time, lose the guilt. It is a tough time, it's okay to not be okay
- Humour
- Have a good routine in place
- Clear work-life boundaries
- Self-care.

How do I cope with the emotional impact of the Covid-19 pandemic?

Over the past few months, we've experienced an unprecedented shift in our way of life due to Covid-19. The Covid-19 pandemic is like nothing that any of us have experienced before. It has presented us with a lot of uncertainty and instability. The emotional reactions that have resulted from the pandemic and the various restriction measures vary from normal to extraordinary. Many people reported a wide range of emotions such as anxiety, fear, depression, frustration, irritability, insomnia, boredom and anger. It is important to be aware of these emotions and take measures to prevent them from snowballing.

These are difficult times and the stress of social isolation, increasing financial uncertainty and a sense of yearning for the lifestyles that we knew before can leave us feeling hopeless. If you are feeling very overwhelmed, if your mood is pervasively low for several days and you are resorting to increasing amounts of substance use to cope with feelings of anxiety and low mood, and if these symptoms are affecting your ability to function at work and at home, please seek the help of a mental health professional. It could be an early sign of a depressive disorder or an anxiety disorder. Depression and anxiety can be treated with a combination of antidepressant medication and therapy, and it is very amenable to treatment. The key is getting help early.

With lockdowns easing around the world and at home, life is slowly resuming some semblance of normalcy. However, it is too soon to say if we will ever go back to the life we knew before the pandemic struck. Coping with the new normal will also bring along its share of challenges. We are affected more than usual when someone sneezes or coughs next to us, outings to the mall or our favourite restaurant will always be weighed against the risk of infection, travelling and holidaying, though increasingly possible, may still not be viable for many of us due to cost, the way we work and study has changed, and the small things that made up our lives are still missing — community sports, meals with big groups of friends; not forgetting also that some of our closed ones, or even favourite establishments did not survive the pandemic.

The first step to dealing with this is to allow yourself to grieve the life that you remember and miss. It is only human to feel this way and you are not alone. And as in any grief reaction, there will be sadness, denial, anger, blame and eventually acceptance of the situation. So, give yourself the time and space to grieve.

Secondly, start by creating a new routine for yourself. Slowly fill the gaps in your old life with something new. If you cannot meet your friends at a cafe, meet them online. If you cannot go to the gym, take up an online fitness class. If your favourite neighbourhood coffee joint has closed, look for a new one to patronise. Get creative and be flexible, the possibilities are endless. The above-mentioned pointers for self-care are even more important to incorporate into your routine now. So focus on your sleep, eat well, and do something relaxing every day. These small changes will reap dividends in time to come.

If you are stuck working at home, try and find things that make you happy during the day. If you train your mind to focus on what goes right in your day, it makes it harder to dwell on what went wrong. This forms the basis of the positive psychology movement. It can even be something as small as the new bag of coffee beans you bought that smells heavenly, admiring the sunrise/sunset or catching up with a friend whom you have not spoken with for some time.

Lastly, be kind to yourself. It is a very difficult situation but do not forget the resources within you that have helped you overcome previous challenges. They will get you through this current situation that you are facing as well. The pandemic will come to an end someday but the resilience forged while battling the emotional aftermath of this extremely stressful period of time will last you a lifetime.

SEXUAL HEALTH

Take Home Points

1. The care for our sexual health encompasses physical aspects, our physiological responses, as well as emotional and mental well-being.
2. To improve the quality of your intimate life — know your own body through the practice of self-pleasure and exploration. Be discerning in obtaining information from the internet, communicate with your partner and work to consciously remove sources of stress in your life.
3. Understanding the differences and triggers for each other allows couples to set up their environment to have a more connected and intimate sex life.
4. If you are feeling immense resistance physically or mentally regarding exploring your sexual wellness, be compassionate with your pace or even work with a sexual wellness expert or therapist.
5. Safety in health, from physical and psychological aspects, are necessary for a thriving sex life and sexuality.

Ms Andrea Tan is a sex, love and relationship coach and sexual wellness educator, and is the founder of Athena Rising.

Introduction

The objectives of this chapter are to build awareness and offer clarity relating to women's sexual health. Sexual health does not just fall under one category of medical care, nor is it limited to the realm of medical care. It encompasses physical aspects, physiological responses, as well as emotional and mental well-being.

What constitutes sexual health for women?

Sexual health, or sexual wellness, essentially covers the areas of sex and sexuality, as well as their connection to the following:

- Relationships & intimacy
- Masturbation & pleasure
- Reproductive health
- Monthly cycle care
- Genital care and sexually transmitted infections (STIs)
- Sexual dysfunctions, e.g., vaginismus, vulvodynia
- Safety, boundaries, consent.

Why is this important to me?

Closing the gap in our knowledge on sexual health is important to our overall physical, emotional and mental well-being, as it can affect our physical and reproductive health, our relationship with our partner, how we view and express our sexuality, and how we experience pleasure.

How do I improve the quality of my sex life and level of intimacy in my relationships?

Know your own body

It is important to know your body, how you respond to various sexual stimulations and arousal techniques, where your erogenous zones are, and your personal preferences. This means taking time to self-pleasure or masturbate. Masturbation allows us to get acquainted with various things like the type of touch we like, how our body responds to arousal, and what arousal feels like for us. It also improves mental and emotional well-being, regulates our body's nervous system and allows for relaxation.

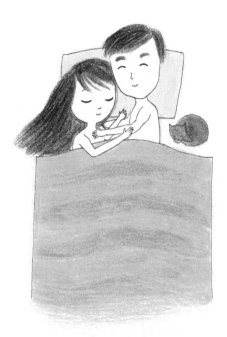

The concept of "sexual brakes and accelerators"[a] provides a simple and pivotal way for couples to share what works for them. It is important to recognise the following:

(i)   Different things or situations (e.g., life stages, times of the day or month, different scents or words or actions) can either enhance our tendency to be turned on or turned off to sex.

---

[a] This idea was referenced in Emily Nagoski's book[1] *Come As You Are*, p. 48, on how the central nervous system (brain and spinal cord) can be described as a series of partnerships of accelerator and brakes ("accelerator" being the sympathetic nervous system and "brake" being the parasympathetic nervous system). To summarise, the sexual accelerator in the "Sexual Excitation System (SES)" receives information about sexually relevant stimuli in the environment which sends signals from the brain to the genitals to indicate turn on; while the sexual brakes constitute the "Sexual Inhibition System (SIS)" by indicating neurological "turn off" stimuli with respect to potential threats in the environment that the brain perceives as turn-offs or a good reason to resist sexual stimulation in a particular moment.

(ii) Everyone has different brakes and accelerators. A life event (e.g., parenthood) may be a brake for one person, and an accelerator for another. Recognising this removes a misunderstanding of your partner's reaction to sex, that it is not personal, but can be attributed to how everyone reacts differently to the same event or situation.

(iii) Unhelpful labels regarding low and high sexual drives should be avoided, e.g., "my husband/wife has a higher sexual drive than me, and we just cannot meet at the same level". It is possible for one person to have more brakes than accelerators, or vice versa. Someone who has more brakes than accelerators, may appear to react more aversely to sexual activity or find it more difficult to experience arousal from their partner.

Understanding the differences and triggers allows each couple to set up necessary conditions in their environment that will support each other, so that they can have a more connected and intimate sex life.

Communicate

Communication is one of the core pillars in maintaining a relationship. Couples are encouraged to schedule time to look specifically at how they communicate with regard to their intimate relationship and sex life.

We consciously learn how to communicate in the corporate world, or how to convey certain ideas in a meeting, or the art of conversation on a first date. The art of communicating intimacy and desires is also a learned skill. Find out if you and your partner have the same understanding of the following: foreplay, great sex, ideal duration of sex, and what words are turn ons/offs. These are essential for couples to navigate sexual conversations effectively. If I do not understand how my partner perceives some of these aforementioned concepts, and I am not able to express my perspectives to my partner, then all the intimate interactions we have end up being based on assumption and guessing — a hotbed for misunderstandings.

Set aside time to communicate with each other, across a series of quality sessions together. Most of these conversations are best discussed before engaging in any intimate activity. Some of these (with enough compassion and gentleness) are even effective in the time right after sex where both partners are usually in a more open state with each other.

Get comfortable to express your needs

We do not always feel comfortable asking for what we want, much less something as intimate and vulnerable about how we want to be touched, or how and when we would like intimacy. Yet, part of building a long-term connected relationship involves communicating specifically about our desires such as how and where we would like to be touched, when we would like to be cuddled, how often we would like to have sex, even when and how we would like to communicate between ourselves and our partners about our sex lives.

Below is a recommended exercise to facilitate the conversation. It might feel rudimentary to speak in such a manner, but it allows both sides to listen to each other without fear of being judged.

Set a timer for each partner to speak. Agree on the context or top 3 conditions that you would need to feel accepted and not judged in the conversation (for instance, eye contact, and questions only at the end of the exercise, and a hug at the end of the exercise). Choose a topic around your sex (or intimate) life that you want to express desires on.

- Partners A and B sit across each other, facing each other with knees touching.
- Partner A (2 mins): "I desire to have some amount of foreplay before we get intimate. I desire to be kissed deeply. I desire to…."
- While Partner A is talking, Partner B looks and nods to acknowledge that he/she is listening.
- When Partner A is done, Partner B expresses what he/she has heard and what he/she would like to do to fulfil Partner A's desires. "I love and accept that you desire this amount of foreplay and to be kissed deeply every day. I would like to be able to provide you this amount of foreplay and to kiss you deeply on the lips at least once a day."
- As Partner B is expressing acknowledgement of Partner A's expressed desires, Partner A experiences receiving the offering from Partner B.
- Once done, both partners can switch positions.
- When both partners are done, do a 10 minute integration. Share with each other about your individual experience in either position, and whether you were triggered, appreciative of what you heard, or if there is anything you want to explore together the next time when you are intimate.

An important note on this exercise is that if you find that both of you or one of you is consistently triggered by an expression of desires or by having to express your own desires, stop the exercise and address the triggers directly. If need be, get professional help to navigate that conversation without allowing triggers to become ways to attack each other or create sources of discontent between the both of you.

Remove sources of stress

While some stress may be sexual accelerators for some people, consistent low-level anxiety conditions usually do not provide a good environment for us to relax, ease into pleasure, slow down and enjoy sex with our partners. While this is seemingly intuitive for those of us working on our overall well-being, conscious efforts to reduce sources of stress directly creates a more conducive environment for us to slow down and appreciate pleasure with our partners. So, identify areas in your schedule, mental stress, physical clutter or digital or scheduling stress that might consume your ability to relax and enjoy the presence of our partner at different times, and especially when we want to get more intimate.

I'm scared and not sure how to masturbate. Is it necessary?

First and foremost, sex and/or masturbation (what I use interchangeably with the term 'self-pleasure') done out of obligation usually does more harm than benefit to our overall well-being and our ability to enjoy pleasure. So, if you are feeling immense resistance physically or mentally regarding masturbation, be compassionate with yourself, you may wish to consider working with a sexual wellness expert or therapist to understand some of the triggers or beliefs that might be preventing you from being intimate with your own body. Usually these stem from fears and beliefs regarding what we judge is right or wrong, or we may be very disconnected from our bodies. Not having experience or not being sure how to masturbate does not mean that something is wrong with you. It is perfectly normal to explore at your own pace, time and only when you are ready.

The benefits of masturbation extend to mental and emotional well-being. As a sexual wellness expert, I often advocate self-pleasure as a part of the self-care routine. The practice of self-pleasure, done consciously with the purpose of allowing the body pleasure, conditions the body to relax and receive pleasure easily, in turn releasing tension held due to emotional or mental stress.

It is also a good way for us to understand our body's responses to the types of arousal and what kind of touch we prefer when being intimate with our partner. This is a great way for us to become comfortable to the sensation of touch. Our fast-paced modern lifestyles can cause us to be disconnected from our bodies and to function predominantly at a more logical, intellectual manner, this is the aspect of ourselves that we need to downplay when having sex or being in a state of pleasure. Part of the ability to relax, be present and open up during sex, or to overall appreciate the intimate experience with our partner is to be less 'in our head' and 'more present in the body'. The practice of self-pleasure teaches this as we practise paying attention to our body cues and feeling arousal versus thinking and conceptualising about it.

I don't feel sexy after having a child. How do I regain my sexuality after childbirth?

Childbirth is physically taxing, and you will need an appropriate amount of time for your body to heal. Ensure that you have adequate rest and a nutritious diet. Regaining your sexuality after childbirth encompasses physical, emotional, and sexual recovery. Physical recovery includes pelvic area muscle recovery or rehabilitation. I use the term 'pelvic area' because this constitutes the muscles that make up our pelvic region, whereas basic Kegel exercises only work the pelvic floor muscles. Emotional recovery includes being able to identify yourself as a sexual being,after childbirth and becoming a mother. Some women feel disconnected from their bodies following childbirth, or they may negatively associate their altered body image with sexuality. Do seek professional help if these feelings persist. Sexual recovery includes the ability of the body to respond to arousal and sexual touch; some of these body cues may have changed during pregnancy and post-partum.

Is orgasm necessary in order to feel pleasure?

The concept of orgasm is the release of the build-up of sexual pleasure, or what some recognise or term as the climax. We do not need to have an orgasm to feel pleasure; often, self-pleasure or sex can still be enjoyable and provide immense pleasure without orgasm. A key thing to note is that the pursuit of an orgasm or the focus on the orgasm, immediately takes away the ability to feel pleasure either in building up or in achieving orgasm. The focus, whether during masturbation or sex, should be to experience the pleasure and its build-up by being present in the moment, instead of waiting and expecting an orgasm.

What has sexual health got to do with my reproductive health?

Care of your genitals and protection against (or early detection and treatment of) sexually transmitted infections (STIs) have direct correlation to our reproductive health. STIs can damage reproductive organs and cause infertility.

Chlamydia and gonorrhoea are preventable causes of pelvic inflammatory disease (PID). If not treated, chlamydia in women can spread to the uterus or fallopian tubes, and cause chronic pain, infertility, and ectopic pregnancy.

On a different note, care of our pelvic and vaginal muscles, allows the uterine and pelvic muscles to withstand the stress of childbirth.

If I do not have period pain, does that mean I do not need to pay attention to my monthly cycles? What is the point of being conscious of my period and monthly cycles?

Even without painful menstrual periods, many of us often experience symptoms during our monthly cycles such as headaches, spotting, diarrhoea, feeling bloated or backaches. On top of that, our body's cervical changes and our body's responses to arousal and ability to produce natural lubrication changes along with the different stages of the monthly cycle.

Understanding how our diet affects these symptoms, and in turn our libido, allows us to work with our cycles rather than feel helpless when something is not right at one point or another of the month.

If you plot in a simple diary, some of the various changes or indicators at different stages of your monthly cycle (follicular, ovulation, luteal, menstrual), you will start to see some patterns emerge. Most phone apps have the ability to track your monthly cycles and calculate these phases based on the information around your first day and the typical duration of each cycle.

In particular, look for the phases where you require some additional lubrication during sex (so you can prepare those beforehand), or where you require a little more sexual stimulation to feel turned on or to reach orgasm. There will be phases (usually the ovulation phase) where you prefer faster, quicker sex with lesser foreplay, or phases where you will prefer the slower type of sensual play (usually the luteal phase). This can allow you to communicate with your partner the changes in your needs so neither of you feel like you are working on your sex life at a different pace.

Do I need soap to keep my vagina/lady bits/vulva clean?

Basic hygiene is part of our self-care routine. Generally, water alone is sufficient. If you prefer to use vaginal soaps, I recommend the ones that are for sensitive skin and without fragrance, and to use them lightly.

Avoid douching the vagina with water or cleaning fluids, as it irritates the vaginal walls and messes with the vaginal pH level. A healthy vaginal pH level is around 3.5 to 4.5. It is slightly acidic, and this is a favourable environment for the healthy flora in the vagina. Changing the vaginal pH level or irritating the vaginal walls, increases the risk of bacterial or yeast infections and may remove the natural mucous on the vaginal walls.

I am worried that I smell below. Is it normal?

Our vaginal discharge and fluids have their own scent. A light tangy, sour or sometimes sweet smell, is generally okay. If the smell is pungent, like rotting fish, do see a doctor to get it checked. Do see a doctor as well if the vaginal discharge appears abnormal, or is associated with a change of colour (grey, yellow or green) and/or consistency (appears chunky or like cottage cheese), or is accompanied by unexplained bleeding, pain or itching, or burning sensation.

How do I know if I may have a STI?

Symptoms of a STI may or may not include: fever, blisters and sores around the genitals or anus, itching around the genitals or anus, rash, unusual vaginal bleeding, pain or irritation during sex, bleeding during sex, lumps or skin growth around the genitals or anus, painful urination, or unusual vaginal discharge.

STI you can also be asymptomatic. If you suspect you might have been exposed to an STI, it is advisable to see a doctor to get it checked and tested.

Is it very disgraceful to go for an STI test?

Understandably, there is a lot of shame and judgement around the topic of STIs. Yet part of our personal health (including sexual health) care is having adequate screening and early detection to allow for suitable and appropriate treatment, and prevent further complications. Doctors are very discreet with STI checks. There are also established home test kits to allow more privacy. Either way, see it as a way to protect yourself and your loved ones, and as a form of general health care.

I have pain at the point of penetration, so I have never experienced penetrative sex. Is there something wrong with me?

Some women experience a condition called vaginismus, essentially (stinging) pain or tension around penetration with a finger or tampon; or tightened vaginal muscles upon penetration. This results in difficult or impossible penetration of the vagina. (Note: there is a condition called vulvodynia where women experience pain in and on the vulva — often unexplained, i.e., tests do not show anything 'wrong' e.g., infections that might be causing the painful reaction.)

It is worth seeing a General Practitioner or gynaecologist to rule out any thrush or bacterial vaginosis, vaginal dryness associated with peri- or post-menopause, or menstrual pain.

If these are ruled out, the tension or pain resulting in difficult or impossible penetration is classified under vaginismus. A few possible underlying reasons include fear, mind-body connection with pain, aversion to sex, and beliefs of past experience regarding sex. It is not correct to assume that vaginismus is caused by something being 'wrong' with you or some sexual trauma. Often there is a mind-body connection with the pain, and a rewiring of the body's connection to pain and sex. For some it could stem from different physiological responses to fear, sex, the idea of penetration or tension. These can be treated with sexual wellness therapists or experts or physios who are trained in pelvic physiotherapy, if the issue stems from pelvic muscle pain and tension.

I have to use lubricant during sex. Is that because I am not normal or not aroused?

No, there is no clear evidence on what constitutes a 'normal' amount of lubrication (vaginal fluids or mucous around the vaginal walls) the body produces. Arousal is also not directly correlated to the amount of natural lubrication our body produces, and it is often referred to as "arousal non-concordance".[b] Our body's reactions and production of natural lubrication varies with different stages of our monthly cycle or our stress levels, given

---

[b] Emily Nagoski summarises the research work that has been done till date over correlation probabilities between arousal, lubrication and causation in Chapter 6 of *Come as You Are*: "Arousal: Lubrication is not Causation".[1]

what we've experienced during the day or what is going on in our lives during that time.

Because sexual stimulation and penetrative sex involve friction, using external lubricants is usually recommended to accommodate more friction that accompanies longer durations of foreplay and/or sexual activity.

What has safety got to do with my sex life or sexuality?

Safety in health, physical and psychological aspects are necessary for a thriving sex life and sexuality.

Safety in the health aspect includes observing genital hygiene practices and preventing exposure to STIs.

Safety in the physical aspect is to ensure safe boundaries when exploring different sexual positions or activities around pain or sensory deprivation, the latter often present in kinky practices. Most kinky activities would require setting up of safe boundaries, safe words, after care and/or agreed upon conditions that allow the physical safety of any participant involved.

Safety in the psychological aspect is whether each partner feels safe enough to be vulnerable, open or receive pleasure through the sexual activity. Part of this psychological safety extends to feeling loved or accepted, without the fear of judgement or shame, and the ability to be vulnerable in an intimate situation with their partner.

Reference

1.   Nagoski E. *Come as You Are*. New York: Simon and Schuster (2015).